One Man's Life-Changing Diagnosis

Navigating the Realities of Prostate Cancer

Craig T. Pynn

D0980773

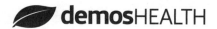

demosHEALTH

Visit our website at www.demoshealth.com

ISBN: 9781936303359
e-book ISBN: 9781617051234

Acquisitions Editor: Noreen Henson
Compositor: diacriTech

Medical information provided by Demos Health, in the absence of a visit with a health care professional, must be considered as an educational service only. This book is not designed to replace a physician's independent judgment about the appropriateness or risks of a procedure or therapy for a given patient. Our purpose is to provide you with information that will help you make your own health care decisions.

The information and opinions provided here are believed to be accurate and sound, based on the best judgment available to the authors, editors, and publisher, but readers who fail to consult appropriate health authorities assume the risk of injuries. The publisher is not responsible for errors or omissions. The editors and publisher welcome any reader to report to the publisher any discrepancies or inaccuracies noticed.

Library of Congress Cataloging-in-Publication Data
CIP data is available from the Library of Congress.

Special discounts on bulk quantities of Demos Health books are available to corporations, professional associations, pharmaceutical companies, health care organizations, and other qualifying groups. For details, please contact:

Special Sales Department
Demos Medical Publishing, LLC
11 West 42nd Street, 15th Floor
New York, NY 10036
Phone: 800-532-8663 or 212-683-0072
Fax: 212-941-7842
E-mail: rsantana@demosmedpub.com

Printed in the United States of America by Bang Printing.
12 13 14 15 / 5 4 3 2 1

This book is dedicated to the memory of my friend, William "Bill" Pantaleo. We shared our deepest feelings and our darkest fears, bonding as only two men with the same advanced disease possibly could. But then this insidious cancer took you so quickly and so ruthlessly at such an early age. Those of us who remain must fight on. One way is by telling our stories. Because that is how the fallen are remembered.

Contents

Foreword   vii

Introduction: An Ordinary Cancer   xi

Acknowledgments   xvii

Part I: Discovery and Diagnosis

  1. Six Scary Words   3

  2. Origins   17

  3. Boarding the Oncology Adventure Ride   35

Part II: Relating to Cancer

  4. Dancing With Cancer   51

  5. Speaking of Cancer   69

  6. Full Speed Ahead   91

Part III: The Other Realities of Prostate Cancer

  7. The Business of Cancer Treatment   109

  8. The Therapeutic Combat Zone   127

  9. But Where Are All the Light Blue Ribbons?   147

Part IV: A Lifetime's Journey

  10. OK, God, So Where Are You, Anyway?   167

  11. Curative, Not Cured: Living With Prostate Cancer   185

Epilogue: The Future of Prostate Cancer   207
Bibliography   215
Index   225

Foreword

I first met Craig almost two years ago, shortly after I was first diagnosed with stage 4 metastatic cancer and started blogging about my own journey. While we've only met once in person at an Us TOO meeting in Chicago, we have grown in the bonds of the prostate cancer brotherhood, becoming strong supporters for each other. In fact, a few months back, he and I made a promise to meet up in a few years, once we both hit the five-year survival mark, to celebrate our victory over a glass of wine with our loving wives and caregivers.

I am honored that he asked me to write the foreword to his book.

The female breast has long been revered in our culture—whether viewed in the context of art, the loving act of motherhood, or a catalyst for sexual attraction. On the other hand, the poor male prostate lies where few want to go, and its important reproductive function is largely underappreciated. As a result, prostate cancer has sat—quite literally—in the shadows.

The psychographics of being male are also a contributor to the problem. As a result, awareness and funding for this disease, which affects more than 16 million men worldwide, lag considerably behind that of breast cancer, despite the fact that—in incidence and mortality—these two cancers are on relatively equal footing. One out of eight American women will be diagnosed with breast cancer in their lifetime while one out of six American men will hear the dreaded words: You have prostate cancer.

This year, nearly 242,000 men will be diagnosed with prostate cancer and more than 28,000 will die from it—that's one death every 18.6 minutes.

Many will point out that the breast cancer movement has had a 10- to 15-year jump on prostate cancer. But the fact remains, our sisters in cancer have done a better job mobilizing and talking about a cancer that greatly affects them. We men tend to avoid talking about our health issue for fear of appearing weak or needy. Worse yet, when it comes to diseases "below the belt," many men fear that those they open up to will assume that some of the possible side effects of treating prostate cancer will undoubtedly have rendered them, in some form or another, less of a man.

The biggest tragedy in this reality is that empathy levels are also lagging. Once diagnosed, many men and their partners or caretakers lack a readily available support system. Often, they embark on their journey with prostate cancer alone, opening the door to feelings of isolation. Worse yet, there are still many men who consciously choose the path of silence and self-exile. It comes as no surprise to me that in my own course of treatment, my urologist, surgeon, radiologist, and oncologist have all peppered their medical interrogations looking for signs of depression. It's a major concern in prostate cancer patients.

I am pleased to observe that as baby boomers age, the shadows are lifting. As a group, boomers are more active consumers of their healthcare, actively researching their conditions and making informed decisions *with* their physicians. The days of one's uncle telling one to not talk about such things or fathers refusing to share their family history with their sons are fading. A new male is emerging. Members of the prostate cancer population are talking more than ever about their concerns and experiences, and Craig is in the vanguard.

With 27 known genotypes or varieties of prostate cancer—some non-life-threatening and others highly aggressive—each diagnosed patient is unique with highly differing prognoses. Yet the fears ignited in us by hearing the "C" word are the same.

Craig's sharing of his experiences with prostate cancer is an honest depiction of personal emotions, including fear, frustration, hope, and the joy of measuring each triumph in his journey.

Before reading the manuscript for this book, I had no idea that my 37 sessions of intensity modulated radiation therapy represented the equivalent of more than 48,000 chest x-rays. But I shouldn't have been surprised. Craig is the same guy who one Saturday morning over coffee and emails helped me figure out how many men on hormone therapy, all hot flashing in unison, it might take to power a small town. His engineering background and patient perspective enable him to break down clinical issues and jargon into easily understandable terms, providing much needed reassurance to patients.

I am grateful to Craig for publishing his story. It is an important read for every patient and their caregivers that will encourage discussion and provide company to families on similar journeys.

An embrace from a fellow member of this fraternal order is like no other. Unspoken, and in a way no other exchange can, it says: *I wish you peace. I wish you strength. I wish you life.* I extend these same wishes to every reader of this book.

Dan Zenka
Los Angeles, California

Dan is a prostate cancer patient and advocate. He blogs regularly about his journey and a wide range of prostate cancer issues at www .mynewyorkminute.org.

He is also senior vice president of communications at the Prostate Cancer Foundation (PCF)—the world's largest private funder of advanced research for prostate cancer cures. Despite having annual prostate cancer screenings for 10 years running, he was diagnosed at age 51 with aggressive prostate cancer just two years after joining PCF. Following a radical prostatectomy, his cancer was upgraded to Stage 4 metastatic disease. He has undergone adjuvant radiation therapy and two years of hormone therapy. Like Craig, he knows well the challenges of running the gauntlet of prostate cancer treatment and is still able to intervene with strong doses of humor as needed.

INTRODUCTION

An Ordinary Cancer

Even though "cancer" and "death" have very different meanings, they became synonymous to me the moment my urologist told me, "You have a nasty cancer." To be sure, cancer is a physical disease. But I have also discovered that it is much more. The tentacles of my disease have reached into every nook and cranny of my being: physical, emotional, psychological, spiritual. Cancer is truly a life-changing diagnosis.

I was 62 years old when I heard the words, "You have cancer." I already knew many people who had been diagnosed with cancer, and several who had died from it. But until that exact moment, cancer was remote, something that happened to other people. But in my urologist's office that cold January morning, I encountered the stark reality of cancer.

Cancer finally became real, because it was happening to me. In the months that followed, the many layers of this disease—some of them quite subtle—began making themselves apparent. There were certainly the clinical realities: diagnosis, treatment, and then living as a cancer survivor. There were the emotional and psychological realities of the disease: cancer's effect on my mental state, and on my personal relationships, notably the one with my wife, Susan. I encountered new spiritual realities, because I believe there is no more potent reminder of one's mortality than hearing the words "You have cancer." Having sat with my friend Bill, first in the hospital, and then in hospice care, watching metastasized prostate cancer take his life, showed me firsthand the real link between cancer and death.

Beyond the personal experiences of prostate cancer, there are the important societal realities. One is the impressive size of the prostate cancer treatment "industry" in the US. Billions of dollars are spent each year—much of them by the federal government—to treat the growing number of men diagnosed each year. As a "leading edge" baby boomer born in 1946, I have come to realize that a growing number of men in my generation will have to navigate the realities of prostate cancer as I have. And the sheer size of this aging generation means that American society will be forced to confront this cancer on a greater scale than it ever has before.

This book is about navigating both the personal and societal realities of prostate cancer.

I am an ordinary man, not so different from the hundreds of thousands of other men who have been diagnosed—or will be diagnosed—with prostate cancer. In many ways, prostate cancer is a very ordinary disease. Yet, it is also extraordinary, for cancer of any kind is a life-altering event. It changes how we see ourselves; how we see others; how we see God. For better or worse, it affects our relationships, and, whether we like it or not, cancer also demands that the people whose lives it invades also form a relationship with it. Even when treatment is completed and cancer is in remission, it is never very far out of sight.

Every few months for the rest of my life, my advanced cancer will require me to re-experience the adrenalin-produced anxiety I often felt as a young person waiting to learn what my future held: that anticipatory dread in the pit of my stomach as I ripped open the envelope containing my SAT scores, the letters of acceptance or rejection from colleges I had applied to, and in one memorable instance, a notice from my draft board that I had been classified fit for military service as the Vietnam War raged. Four decades later, it's the envelope containing the results of my latest blood test that produces the same foreboding. Has my PSA level remained undetectable? Or is it rising? Because if it's rising, there is the rising probability that my cancer has returned.

Prostate cancer (like every other cancer) pushes ordinary people into extraordinary circumstances. Ordinary men—and the wives, sons, daughters, and partners who love them—must deal with the reality that inside an obscure organ they've rarely thought about, rogue cells are multiplying. Worse, the battle is occurring at the epicenter of a man's sexual identity. And while dealing with this bad news, these ordinary men and their caregivers must summon the will to navigate the labyrinth of modern American medicine. Prostate cancer patients will submit to seemingly endless and invasive tests. Then, they must choose from a confusing array of treatment options, or possibly decide to forego any treatment at all. Too often, this crucial decision must be made with inadequate medical guidance. Then, these men must endure the treatment itself—sometimes for years—with all the accompanying short- and long-term consequences. Prostate cancer patients and their loved ones will have to deal with the reality of disease while still attempting to live their daily lives. In too many cases, they will struggle to keep working in order to avoid financial catastrophe for their families.

Even when treatment is complete, there is the aftermath: recovery and lingering side effects. Some men deal with incontinence. Many more cope with impotence. For men on hormone therapy, there are the physical, mental, and emotional stresses of living without testosterone. And for many of us, there is a lingering "overhang": the very real possibility that the cancer will return. While there is plenty of literature and medical advice for dealing with the physical challenges of prostate cancer, there are few books that address its substantial emotional and psychological costs.

The term "cancer survivor" is ubiquitous in American society. In the midst of cancer's many fundraising efforts, awareness campaigns, and media stories, cancer survivors are celebrated as local heroes. But what is it *really* like to be a "survivor," living with the reality of a cancer like mine, that will never be definitively cured, but can only be treated and managed? This question is at the heart of my personal story and the stories of many men with prostate cancer, especially those of us with advanced versions of this disease.

While each man's prostate cancer diagnosis is an extraordinary event in his life, in statistical terms, prostate cancer is actually quite common. As if offering proof of its ordinariness, I discovered shortly after being diagnosed that most everyone I knew had a husband, father, grandfather, brother, uncle, cousin, or friend who had been diagnosed with prostate cancer. After skin cancer, prostate cancer is the most widespread carcinoma among men in the United States. One in six men in the US will be diagnosed with prostate cancer at some point during his lifetime.

Yet, despite its ubiquity, prostate cancer has yet to reach the level of public awareness of some other cancers. Women have done a superb job communicating with the public about the need for more screening, research, and treatment to cure breast cancer. The pink ribbons and pink-themed products that proliferate every October—Breast Cancer Awareness Month—are a testimony to their successful efforts. But few people know that September is Prostate Cancer Awareness month, or that light blue ribbons symbolize the struggle against prostate cancer in the same way that pink ribbons represent the fight against breast cancer.

Given this contrast in public visibility, one could easily conclude that the number of women diagnosed with breast cancer each year in the US must be far greater than the number of men diagnosed with prostate cancer. Actually, the numbers are roughly equal at slightly over two hundred thousand each. The reasons behind this "awareness gap" are complex. Much of the disparity lays in behavioral differences between men and women. This reality is worth exploring.

Also worth investigating are the historical underpinnings of prostate cancer diagnosis and treatment in America. Where does this cancer come from? How did it end up with so many treatment regimens? What are its worrying demographic implications? Why are African Americans more likely to get prostate cancer than Whites, who in turn are more likely to be diagnosed than Asians and Hispanics? What are some of the back room treatment controversies within the medical community? Is screening for prostate cancer via the PSA test essential to public health or the easy path to needless overtreatment? How do the dynamics of the multi-billion dollar prostate cancer industry affect patients? Is increasingly expensive treatment technology on a collision course with economic reality as more men are diagnosed with this cancer? Are government bodies, medical practices, hospitals marketing robotic surgery, radiation oncology centers, and pharmaceutical companies acting altruistically, or are there other financial motivations at work?

Behind all the historical, medical, and political questions, however, the central priority is clear: the individual man who has prostate cancer. Stories written by men who have prostate cancer are scarce. Many men just want to get the disease behind them and not talk about it. For these men, prostate cancer is just a question of being diagnosed, getting treated, and moving on without looking back. But, as I discovered, it is not always that simple. Dealing with prostate cancer is not just about treating a medical condition. It is often about far more than that.

Plenty of books discussing this cancer's clinical aspects already exist. Most of them provide crucial information about a cancer that can take an enormous variety of forms and has a dizzying array of treatment methods. Also, there are numerous books brimming with advice about what to do, or what not to do, when receiving a prostate cancer diagnosis. These books have titles that employ militaristic words like "conquering," "beating," and "surviving."

But there are fewer first-person stories that describe a prostate cancer patient's life-changing journey from diagnosis through treatment into the new reality of cancer survivor. Scarcer still are personal accounts that describe a man's thoughts and feelings along the way: what it's like to be probed, biopsied, injected, scanned, radiated, medicated, or operated upon; what it's like to deal with the effects of treatment; and perhaps, eventually, to deal with the reality of his cancer's recurrence.

To weave my personal story into the larger social realities of prostate cancer is the objective of this book. More importantly, however, I chose to share my story to help the man who one day will hear, or perhaps has already heard, the same scary words that I did: "You have prostate cancer."

As this newly diagnosed man and his family struggle to understand his diagnosis, they might want to read about the experiences and feelings of a man who once faced what they are now facing. They may want to hear how the issue is often not just "conquering" or "beating" cancer, but coming to terms with it. This is the story not just of my diagnosis and treatment, but also of how untrammeled emotions—and fears—invaded my life at unexpected moments. How the treatments aimed at eradicating cancer sometimes seemed almost worse than the cancer itself. How cancer affected my relationships with other people, especially my wife. How it felt when the euphemistically named "hormone therapy" turned me into a eunuch. How it is to continue living under the "overhang" of cancer's recurrence for the remainder of my life. How it all seems so unfair, but at the same time how this disease has helped me grow emotionally and spiritually.

This book is written for that one newly diagnosed man who, by reading my story, will discover that he does not have to make this journey alone.

Acknowledgments

Cancer is not a journey to be made alone. Since first hearing the scary words, "You have a nasty prostate cancer," I am immensely thankful that I have not had to hike this long trail by myself.

First, I am grateful for the wisdom and expertise of my doctors, urologist Dr. Brian Hopkins and radiation oncologist Dr. Vince Massullo. Both have kindly given their permission to appear as themselves in this book, and you will come to know them in these pages as they provided guidance and encouragement, not to mention expert treatment. I'm thankful, too, to the other medical professionals I have encountered along the way, especially those at Pacific Urology and the John Muir Radiation Oncology Center, whose expert hands and caring hearts have helped make the seemingly endless trek through cancerland bearable. You will meet some of them in this book, too, although I have identified them only by their first names.

Then, there is the little community that surrounded Susan and me with care and love through the months of diagnosis and treatment: Lin and Dennis Ashlock; Chuck and Jenny Hammond; and Dave and Nancy Pierce. Your longstanding friendship is a jewel beyond price. And to the men of Hubcaps: you know who you are. I am privileged to be among a group of men every Friday morning, who laugh together, challenge each other, and above all, care deeply for one another as they demonstrate their faith day after day through prayer and generous acts of love.

To son Geoff, daughter Elisabeth, daughter-in-law Roxanne, and son-in-law Jacob: Your concern, caring, encouragement, and passion have been as powerful a medicine as any clinical treatment. To grandsons Ivan and Jens, and granddaughter Lydia: You are the light of my life and the consummate motivation for me to beat this disease, and to be able to watch you grow and mature.

Writing a book about cancer requires a small village of willing participants. Profound gratitude goes first to my daughter-in-law, Roxanne Willis, herself a gifted writer and author, for her research, her perceptive editing, and her concision. Without Roxanne's ability to refashion my prose succinctly and stylishly, you would have a more difficult time reading this book.

Thank you, Yvonne Hanson, for your valuable insights into the psychology of disease, and for helping me put words to what before was only a vague sense that we men deal with cancer quite differently than women do.

Thanks, too, for the patience and invaluable insights of my four "trusted readers," Ann Clausen, Terry Drula, Tim Johnson, and Ken Neff. Each of you grappled courageously with early drafts with unfailing good humor and, above all, enormously helpful corrections and suggestions.

I am deeply indebted to Noreen Henson at Demos Health Publishing for finding merit in my story and overseeing its transformation into tangible reality.

None of these people is responsible for any errors in this book. That responsibility is mine alone.

Finally, gratitude beyond words to my wife Susan. You have shown in your loving (and patient!) ways that notwithstanding our respective diseases, we are on this journey together for keeps and that in spite of ourselves, we are indeed "the big door prize."

PART I
DISCOVERY AND DIAGNOSIS

ONE

Six Scary Words

ENCOUNTERING A NEW REALITY

On a cool November morning in Walnut Creek, California, I waited in a small exam room to see Dr. Brian Hopkins. Just as with my last appointment with him seven years ago, he was running late. The sterile-feeling room lacked any old magazines, and I had forgotten to bring a book with me. The only available distraction was a poster featuring a full-color cutaway drawing of the male genitourinary anatomy.

"Clever marketers, these urologists," I thought. "What a great name for a urology practice. Pacific Urology—it makes one think of the Pacific Ocean and palm trees waving gently in the warm sea breeze. Calming and relaxing."

Which was not exactly how I felt at the moment. Instead, I could barely suppress the surge of nervousness that always accompanies me to these doctor visits. I was naturally dreading the probing around "down under" that accompanies any visit to the urologist.

"Hi, Craig," Dr. Hopkins said, as he strode into the room with a friendly smile and handshake. He was about the same height as I, although in better physical shape, looking as energetic and youthful as when I last saw him. "Good to see you again. It's been a while."

"It certainly has," I replied with the packaged cheerfulness I've always tried to summon in these doctor-patent situations. The professional pleasantries thus completed, I began to explain why I had come to see him. Dr. Hopkins took notes on his clipboard as he listened to me explain why I was there. My story began about two months earlier.

The steady rain that had been beating down on the Chicago suburbs for three days had finally ended. My wife, Susan, and I were completing a five-day visit with our son, daughter-in-law, and two young grandchildren. This morning we would start the final leg of our leisurely cross-country drive from our home in the San Francisco Bay Area to our vacation home in Massachusetts. There, we planned to enjoy autumn in New England, as we often did, preferring the crisp days and cold nights of Massachusetts to the arid fall heat of northern California.

It was barely light enough to see the face of my watch reading 5:30 a.m. as I climbed out of bed. Like most men past a certain age, I headed straight to the bathroom. Urinary relief achieved, I was shocked to see several reddish clots in the toilet bowl. Looking up, the mirror over the sink revealed a black and blue mark stretching from my left kidney area to my navel, a dramatic souvenir from a household accident that had occurred three days ago in this very bathroom. While attempting to drill into a stubborn ceramic tile in the shower, I had slipped on a wet spot on the floor. My fall was brought to an abrupt and painful halt by the aluminum track of the glass shower door mounted on the tub rim.

"There must be some internal bleeding from that fall," I self-diagnosed. "I'll need to get that looked at when we get to Massachusetts."

As we drove eastward that morning, we discovered that recent rainstorms had flooded roadways everywhere, forcing us into a time-consuming detour at the Illinois-Indiana border. Morning coffee filled my bladder as we sat in the excruciatingly slow-moving traffic. At last, relief was in sight. A McDonald's loomed into view. Pulling into the parking lot, I lost no time in finding the men's room.

The sight in the urinal was not encouraging. There was blood everywhere, including several sizable clots. My stomach lurched.

I knew I should really have this checked out—and soon. But we were now in an unfamiliar part of Indiana. The idea of finding an emergency room (ER) here, of all places, was unappealing at best. Electing to exercise my male prerogative to tough it out, I decided not to mention my situation to Susan. I would tell her later when we were closer to Massachusetts. I even naively hoped that this problem might just go away by itself.

Withholding information from my wife was not normal behavior on my part, especially about something that felt so serious. After nearly forty years of marriage, there were few secrets remaining between us. There was something about her habitual honesty that inevitably compelled me to come clean with her, and I knew that I would be telling her about my condition soon. But to tell her right now would lead to her insistence on finding a hospital immediately, here in the Indiana outback, and then who knows how long we would be stuck waiting in an emergency room. There was no pain associated with the blood, so I was able to continue driving, trying to block the scary situation from my mind.

We made slow progress heading east that day. At rest stops along the Indiana Toll Road and the Ohio Turnpike, I headed nervously to the men's room, each time hoping that what I had seen earlier might just disappear. But there was always more blood.

Finally, we pulled into the parking lot of a hotel abutting the New York Thruway, exhausted by a long day of driving. As we lay in bed just before drifting off, I steeled my courage and said, "Uh, I have a problem, I think. I've been peeing some blood today."

Susan shifted instantly from sleepiness to high alert. "What did you say?"

"Well, you know that fall I took on Friday, and the big black and blue mark I got? I think I must have injured something internally. I should probably see a doctor when we get to Massachusetts."

"How come you didn't say anything earlier? You need to have this checked out."

"Well," I fudged, omitting mention of the traces of blood I had seen in the early morning at our son's home, "It really didn't show up till we were in Indiana this morning, and I did not want to be stuck in an ER in some little rural town for who knows how long."

"You really should have told me before this. This is significant. You need to get it looked at."

"I know. I'm sorry I didn't tell you earlier. But it's bleeding less now, so I think things are improving."

"We are headed to the ER as soon as we get to Massachusetts."

I could tell from the quiver in her voice that Susan's feelings were oscillating between anger and worry. I was pretty sure that worry was the dominant emotion. I was worried, too, but didn't want to add to her anxiety. It had been a long and stressful day, and neither of us had enough energy for a prolonged discussion, or worse yet, a fight. Soon enough, we fell asleep.

When we arrived in Massachusetts the following day, there was no longer any blood in my urine. Only the black and blue mark remained. I argued that it probably wasn't necessary to go to the emergency room after all, but Susan insisted, "You really need to have this looked at."

At an earlier point in our relationship, this disagreement could have led to an argument. Today, however, was different. I was fearful. Clearly, something had gone wrong inside me. This time I only made a half-hearted attempt to avoid a doctor's visit. Susan's logic ultimately prevailed, and we headed to the local hospital.

An emergency room is hardly the ideal venue for diagnosing the root causes of symptoms that have vanished. But given our insurance situation, it was nearly impossible to get an appointment with a primary care doctor in Massachusetts. And since the Commonwealth lacks the freestanding "urgent care" clinics we were accustomed to in northern California, we had no choice but to turn to the expensive inefficiencies of the ER.

After I had gone through the usual opening ceremonies of an emergency room visit—putting on a gown, getting my blood pressure and pulse taken, having an IV inserted, and donating a urine sample—Susan and I settled in the curtained cubicle to wait. After showing the doctor my purpled abdomen and offering my "it must be an internal injury" theory, he ordered a CT scan.

After the CT scan was finished, we waited for another hour. Finally, the doctor reappeared with all of my test results in hand. "You have a urinary tract infection," he announced. "And the CT scan is clear. It doesn't show any sign of injury. You should set up an appointment with a urologist." He proceeded to give me a prescription for an antibiotic and handed me a CD with the CT scan images on it.

I am one of those relatively few men who have experienced a urinary tract infection (UTI) every two or three years for most of my adult life. But this certainly did not feel like a classic UTI, nor had I had blood in my urine with previous infections. This time there had been no pain, just blood, and even that had disappeared by now. Rather than challenge the diagnosis, however, I gratefully opted to leave the ER. So I quickly took my prescription and disk, dressed, and we left.

However, the ambiguous outcome of the emergency room visit did not satisfy me. I was left with a nagging suspicion that the medical staff believed something more serious was going on, and the real problem had been papered over with a UTI diagnosis. I also believed that the medical team had simply ignored my theory of a fall-related injury as the ranting of a misinformed layperson. But I knew full well that my self-diagnosis had inconsistencies. Why did the bleeding not start until three days after the fall? Why hadn't the CT scan revealed any sign of internal injury under the black and blue on my abdomen? Because I wanted desperately to believe I was okay, however, I continued to hypothesize that my bathroom fall was the cause of the bleeding.

Since I was unable to set up an appointment during the six weeks we were in Massachusetts, I made a date to see a urologist after we returned to California. This was a physician I already knew, Dr. Brian Hopkins, who had treated me for a urinary tract infection more than seven years ago in 2001. And this is how I ultimately ended up in this exam room at Pacific Urology, telling my story to him.

Dr. Hopkins listened patiently, nodding, and taking notes. "Let's take a look at the CT scan," he said. After a few moments of scrolling through the scan's images on his computer, he concluded that the scans were good quality, and like the ER doctor, he did not see any obvious sign of fall-induced injuries. My "internal bleeding" theory began to seem much less credible—even to me.

The list of possible diagnoses was starting to narrow, which made me increasingly nervous. Prior to my appointment, Susan and I had discussed some vague possible diagnoses. By the time

I saw Dr. Hopkins, the bleeding was in the past, and I assumed it was not going to start up again. Because of this, I managed to persuade Susan there was no reason for her to accompany me on the tiring 50-mile round trip from our home to Pacific Urology.

No man's visit to the urologist is complete without the obligatory digital rectal exam (DRE), and as I had anticipated, Dr. Hopkins did not disappoint me. "Let's feel your prostate," he said.

After I assumed the position known to most men over the age of fifty or so, the doctor's latex-gloved finger probed, stopped, and probed some more. He seemed to linger where other doctors had efficiently gotten in and back out again.

"Uh, oh," he said. "Bad prostate."

The "bad prostate" pronouncement came as a shock. That there might be a problem with my prostate had not crossed my mind. I knew my prostate was enlarged, but the "uh, oh" had a distinctly ominous tone to it. I suddenly feared that Dr. Hopkins's statement might mean something serious. But even so, I didn't immediately think of cancer. At my physical exam eight months earlier, my primary care physician performed a DRE and told me that my prostate felt normal. "Somewhat enlarged, but nothing out of the ordinary," she had assured me. And my prostate-specific antigen (PSA) numbers—which become elevated when a man has prostate cancer or any number of other prostate conditions—had remained steady at around 1.5 for the past seven years. The current medical wisdom was that a PSA value below 4.0 was "normal." (I would learn later that what should be considered a "normal" PSA is the subject of much debate among medical experts.)

Dr. Hopkins, unaware of my growing anxiety, continued in his professional manner, "We need to schedule a prostate biopsy. And we'll need to do a cystoscopy, too."

The biopsy was scheduled in the busy run-up to Christmas. "What a terrific Christmas present," I thought. "A needle biopsy through my rectum. I can hardly wait." During the intervening month between the discovery of my "bad prostate" and the biopsy, I reflected occasionally on what Dr. Hopkins's statement might really signify. The possibility that cancer could be the diagnosis finally entered my conscious mind. But I successfully suppressed these thoughts as quickly as they arose.

In mid-December, I was back in an exam room at Pacific Urology, this time curled up on my left side, naked from the waist down, my modesty barely preserved by a flimsy paper drape. A prostate biopsy is an uncomfortable but bearable procedure, during which the doctor uses a spring-loaded, needle-tipped instrument to remove small core samples of prostate cells, which are sent to the pathologist for analysis. Typically, the urologist removes anywhere from eight to twelve samples from various regions of the prostate gland. A prostate "needle biopsy" is the only reliable method to assess cellular conditions inside the prostate—and the only way to determine whether or not cancer is present.

Guided by the ultrasound probe inserted into my rectum, Dr. Hopkins worked on capturing twelve samples of my prostate—six from each side of the gland—by repeatedly squeezing the trigger on his trusty spring-loaded apparatus. A lidocaine-dampened sting accompanied the "snap" of the spring releasing—a sound similar to the type of old-fashioned cap gun I proudly owned when I was about eight years old. As he worked, we chatted amiably about Susan's and my peripatetic life divided between California and Massachusetts. The otherwise-pleasant conversation was interrupted periodically by the snapping sound and the momentary sting deep inside my pelvis. Obviously experienced at this, Dr. Hopkins completed the biopsy in less than ten minutes.

"OK, we're set. I'll send these off to the lab and we'll have the results in a couple of weeks," he said. "That's a little longer than usual because of the holidays."

"That's fine," I replied. "I'm perfectly happy to enjoy Christmas in the meantime."

A week following the biopsy, Susan and I flew east to join our children and grandchildren for an actual white Christmas at my son's home in Illinois, now personally infamous to me as the site of that tumble onto the bathtub rim. At my daughter-in-law's request—and with a sense of gratifying justice—I dismantled the tub enclosure, happy to dispose of the sharp-edged aluminum track that had led, however indirectly, to a prostate biopsy.

Perhaps it was being geographically close to the site of my fall, but a premonition lurked during this Christmas visit: Maybe September's symptoms really meant something more significant than a simple injury from a bathroom accident. What did Dr.Hopkins suspect? What did he already know that he wasn't telling me? Cancer? But my thoughts remained abstract, oddly free of emotion—something like, "Ah, yes, cancer. Well, that could be an interesting medical situation."

I had a hazy memory of reading something about the "seven warnings signs of cancer," one of which was blood in the urine. But I quickly decided that these warning signs were obsolete, coming from the dark ages before PSA tests. And my PSA level was normal anyway—and had been normal for the past seven years. The happy distraction of my grandchildren celebrating Christmas quickly pushed the dark thoughts out of my mind. Surely, I rationalized, I was just fine.

As it turned out, Pacific Urology had to reschedule the cystoscopy appointment from early January to later in the month. That was fine with me. Several of my previous UTIs had led to cystoscopies, and I was in no rush to hear the doctor once again say "You may experience some momentary discomfort" when what I really felt was pain. As the calendar moved to the appointed day, I suspected that the results of the biopsy might be back from the lab by now. But no one had called to discuss the results yet. So, choosing to believe that "no news is good news," I decided that the biopsy results were probably normal.

Arriving for the cystoscopy, I was again covered from the waist down by the paper drape, this time while lying uncomfortably on my back on the too-short exam table. After the doctor's assistant administered the lidocaine anesthetic to numb the relevant body parts, I lay there, waiting for my urinary tract to be explored with the aid of fiber optics. After sufficient time had passed for the drug to kick in, Dr. Hopkins appeared, and with his usual cheerful aplomb, he grasped the business end of the probe and began the task at hand. A "cysto," in the urological jargon, involves inserting a lighted, flexible fiber optic tube somewhat analogous to a plumber's "snake" up the urethra and into the bladder. The fiber optics are connected to a magnifying "scope," which allows the doctor to examine the inside of the urethra and bladder.

Suffice it to say, a probe squeezed down the full length of the male urethra creates a sense of alien invasion. It is not painful (the drugs have taken care of that), but there are odd sensations that do not occur naturally. Skilled urologists are usually quite efficient, taking a thorough but speedy look at the interior of the bladder and urethra before removing the cystoscope, providing instant relief. This time, however, he kept the probe lingering uncomfortably inside me, obviously examining something quite carefully.

"I see a lesion in your urethra that I want to check out further," he stated matter-of-factly. "We'll need to schedule a urethral biopsy."

"Uh, oh," I thought. "He's starting to take this situation too seriously. Something must not be quite right."

Finally he withdrew the scope. And as if on cue, his assistant knocked on the door and appeared with a paper in her hand. "Here is the lab report you asked for, Doctor." Tossing caution to the wind, little caring that I was still lying half-naked on the exam table covered by a now-crumpled paper drape, the question that up to now had been so easy to ignore for so many months spilled forth: "What does it say?"

"You have a nasty prostate cancer," he answered.

Six scary words. Nine syllables. I looked around. The small exam room seemed to lose what little color it had. A gray haze of "this really isn't happening to me" washed out all other thoughts.

Much like my urinary tract, my comfortable world—shrouded in denial for so long—had suddenly been invaded by an alien presence.

IS CANCER DIFFERENT?

Like almost every other member of the baby boomer generation, I remember exactly where I was and what I was doing—and even what the weather was like—on November 22, 1963, when I heard that President Kennedy was shot. Similarly, most Americans remember their exact position in space and time when they witnessed the horrible events of September 11, 2001. People also tend to remember the details of major life events, such as weddings and the births of children. January 22, 2009—the day I heard "you have prostate cancer"—joins my short list of unforgettable moments. I believe that every person who receives a cancer diagnosis never forgets the precise time, location, and circumstances in which they first heard the news. Perhaps this type of "memory freeze" occurs whenever someone is diagnosed with a significant disease. I cannot know for sure, because until this January morning, I had escaped other serious diagnoses like diabetes or heart disease. But however similar it might be to other diseases, I think there is something uniquely frightening about cancer. In the days following my diagnosis, I reflected on why the word *cancer* created so much fear in me—and in other people.

The Roman physician and philosopher Galen (AD 129–200) is credited with naming breast tumors whose shape resembled the claws of a crab. In the style of many Roman academics of his era, he chose to give his discovery a Greek name, *karkinos*, meaning, "crab." Ultimately though, it was the word "cancer," which is the Latin word for "crab," that became the standard term in English and the Romance languages. Regardless of the language chosen, "crab" is an appropriate name for a disease that is characterized by its ability to hold on so tightly to its sufferer.

Cancer and death have been closely associated since the disease was first named and understood. This connection makes sense: Until recently, cancer *was* a death sentence, a disease whose end stages were invariably accompanied by unbearable pain. Modern therapies have substantially reduced the mortality rates of widespread cancers such as breast cancer, prostate cancer, and skin cancer. Still, as James Patterson argues, a deep fear and the distinct possibility of death continue to lurk in the phrase, "He (or she) has cancer."

This same feeling of cultural dread does not seem to accompany other diseases that are as potentially deadly as cancer. Phrases like "He has heart disease" do not seem to carry the same certain specter of death, even though heart disease kills more people each year in the United States than cancer.

Well-publicized horror stories about cancer, especially those involving Hollywood celebrities, are often touted in supermarket tabloids, reinforcing the popular idea that cancer inevitably causes death. We unconsciously conclude that cancer treatment may slow a person's demise, but still, deep down we believe he or she will probably die from it. Unfortunately, for some cancers, such as those in the lung, pancreas, or liver, this is still often true.

The fact that cancer arises from mutations of existing cells in the body underscores its dreadfulness.

> Cancer is the uncontrolled growth of abnormal cells in the body. Cancerous cells are also called malignant cells. A *carcinogen* is a substance capable of causing cancer.
>
> *Source: National Cancer Institute*

There are abundant external causes of cancer. Cancer itself causes cells in our body to rebel against the proper structure and functioning of some previously healthy organ. The fact that cancer *grows inside us* taps directly into many of our deepest fears. When we have cancer, we have a monster living within us. Worse, many cancers grow quietly, unnoticed until sometimes it is too late. My own cancer tricked my PSA response mechanism, managing to remain undetected before it finally produced a visible symptom—blood in my urine. Even then I had felt nothing: no pain, no discomfort.

There are about 200 different types of cancer, some truly dreadful and incurable, others far less so. Cancer may affect any of the 60 different body organs. And there are about 210 known cell types in the human body, any of which may become cancerous. But not all cancers are created equal. So, we need to be careful not to assume that all cancers carry with them an automatic death sentence.

Still, the idea of malignancy seems built into the very word itself. Even if "cancer" meant "beautiful, fragrant flower," it is not a pleasant-sounding word, with its hard-edged first syllable and a sibilant "s" on the second. Its more technical term, "carcinoma," derived directly from the Greek, sounds even more threatening.

More than any other disease, cancer is seen as an enemy to be conquered. We "fight" and "battle" cancer. Patients being treated are often called "warriors," those who make it through treatment are cancer "survivors." The United States has been engaged in a "war on cancer" for forty years. We do not hear of wars on heart disease or Parkinson's with anything near the public fervor that "battling cancer" or "conquering cancer" generates.

As I struggled to absorb Dr. Hopkins's bad news in the exam room, I felt only cancer's overwhelming malevolence. When I heard him say, "You have a nasty prostate cancer," my mind instantly appended "… and that means you're toast, buddy." As I subsequently found out, prostate cancer is one of the most survivable cancers. But at that moment any hint of optimism had been snuffed out by a very real dread. The word *cancer* had brought its associations with death, and I felt all the dread and fear that the diagnosis carries with it.

Each year, the same scary words that I heard—"You have prostate cancer"—are spoken to approximately 200,000 American men—more than 500 men each day of the year. According to the National Cancer Institute, the number of men diagnosed with prostate cancer each year is about equal to the number of women diagnosed with breast cancer. Add to this the estimated two million prostate cancer survivors in the United States, and it is little wonder that almost everyone knows a man who has had prostate cancer. Because of these large numbers, much is known about prostate cancer, but as we shall see, it has numerous variations. Urologists and oncologists generally encounter few surprises when diagnosing and treating it, although, as it turned out in my own case, there were a few unexpected twists, even for my highly experienced urologist.

In a country that is now supposedly supportive of full gender equality, prostate cancer is one of the few remaining "men's only" clubs. Famous survivors of prostate cancer include actor Robert De Niro; politicians Rudy Giuliani, John Kerry, and Bob Dole; Bishop Desmond Tutu; and Andy Grove, a founder of the semiconductor manufacturer Intel. Many of these cases, like Rudy Giuliani's, have received worldwide publicity. Others, like Bishop Desmond Tutu's, are relatively unknown. The hopeful commonality among these men is that they have resumed active lives as prostate cancer survivors.

Each man has demonstrated that, while prostate cancer is a major life event, it is a challenge that can be met and overcome.

In the months following my diagnosis, my spirits were lifted by the example set by these men and also by the data showing the survivability of prostate cancer. Nevertheless, deep inside my brain the words *cancer* and *death* remained locked in a grim embrace.

After Dr. Hopkins left the exam room the morning of my diagnosis, I remained in a mental fog as I dressed. The reality of my cancer had been spoken aloud, but I was far from understanding what this all really meant. American culture emphasizes youth and virility, underscored by the omnipresent commercials on television that promote virility insurance in the form of medications, promising "You'll be ready when she's ready." Men are usually quite happy to describe their athletic or sexual prowess to one another. But prostate cancer is the antithesis of sexual prowess and virility. The widely known side effects of prostate cancer treatment—impotence and incontinence—affect a man at the ground zero of his masculinity. These realities of prostate cancer were only beginning to dawn on me.

There was another reason for my mental fog. On the day the scary words were spoken, my ability for rational thought was supplanted by adrenaline-driven fear. There are a number of ways to be driven into a state of shock. For me, hearing "You have a nasty prostate cancer" was one of them. It would take a while for mental clarity to return.

TWO

Origins

REFLECTIONS ON A BIOPSY

If real life worked like the ideal scenarios described in many cancer advice books, right after hearing that I had prostate cancer I would have asked my doctor to see a copy of my biopsy report. We would have then calmly reviewed its contents together. I would have posed intelligent questions that would have elicited further important details about my diagnosis. By the end of the meeting, I would have felt like a fully informed patient, calmly accepting the diagnosis, and ready to reflect placidly on the logical treatment alternatives confronting me.

But after I heard those six scary words, "You have a nasty prostate cancer," this ideal scenario was not remotely close to how events played out. After I eventually summoned the will to get dressed and meet Dr. Hopkins in his office, I heard only every third or fourth word that he spoke, comprehending little more than the fact that I had cancer, and apparently there were some pills I should start taking. Simply acting composed at the Pacific Urology checkout desk as the medical administrator filled out my paperwork took enormous effort. Remaining upright as I walked, clutching the lab test papers in my sweaty hand consumed the totality of my available brainpower. My bewildered emotional state trumped any possibility for clear thought. In the thirty minutes following Dr. Hopkins's pronouncement of my diagnosis, I managed to skip just about every rational step that the cancer advice books direct newly diagnosed cancer patients to take.

One of the recommendations I did not follow that day was to ask for a copy of my biopsy report. Given my emotional state and my profound ignorance of prostate cancer, I would probably have understood little of it anyway. As the reality of cancer began to sink in, I actually forgot all about the pathology report—that fateful piece of paper that Dr. Hopkins's assistant had delivered to him in the exam room. I simply took my doctor at his word that I had an aggressive form of prostate cancer. The writers of cancer advice books would surely have frowned on my naïve willingness to accept this important fact based solely on one doctor's declaration.

> You should have a copy of your pathology report. If you forgot to take it with you, call and ask your doctor for a copy.

It took more than a year for me to realize that I had never looked at the original biopsy report. When I finally requested a copy from Pacific Urology, they quickly produced one for me. The four-page color report was impressive to look at, suggesting it was quite expensive to produce. At the top left of the first page were my name and identifying information, laying to rest my occasional fantasy that this was all a big mistake, that my results had been mixed up with someone else's.

A full color picture of one of the stained specimens on the first page was labeled, "Adenocarcinoma, Right Lateral Apex." In color and texture it resembled a close-up of the Italian dry salami that is a delicatessen staple in the San Francisco Bay Area. I only needed to search for a few minutes on the web to find photomicrographs of the different grades of prostate cancers. The colored photo on my biopsy report exactly matched the photo on my computer screen labeled "example of Gleason 4 carcinoma."

Staring at the image of my Right Lateral Apex Adenocarcinoma created a jabbing sensation inside my brain. Here was a photograph of my own flesh taken from deep inside my body—and it was cancerous. For the first time, more than a year after my diagnosis, I had visible evidence of what all the fuss was about. What had been cancer in the abstract was now cancer in reality. I was staring my opponent in the face.

To the immediate right of the photo on the biopsy report was a stylized map of the prostate, divided into neat squares: three in the right-hand column were labeled "Right Lat Base," "Right Lat Mid," and "Right Lat Apex." The three on the left-hand side were similarly labeled. Each of these six squares represented an area of prostatic territory from which Dr. Hopkins had extracted two samples, a total of twelve core samples in all. Inside each of the six squares on the report was a small pie chart. Each pie represented the percentage malignancy for that particular neighborhood of my prostate. The percentage of malignancy on each pie chart was indicated in red. The more red in the chart, the more cancerous the sample. Three of the pies were almost completely filled in with red, indicating they were 80 percent cancerous, two were marked 70 percent, and one was marked a relatively modest 40 percent. All that red; all that cancer.

The report continued with a section titled, "Prostate, Needle Biopsies," describing the detailed analysis of each of the twelve specimens examined by the pathologist. An example entry, again printed in capital letters, using the same the dramatic red ink of the pie charts, read: "Right Lat Mid: Adenocarcinoma (Gleason score 4 + 4 = 8) involving 80% of the specimen (2 of 2 cores contain cancer)." This list continued through all twelve sample specimens, eleven of them printed in red capital letters. Only one of the entries, named "Right Lat Base," provided some visual relief from the insistent red capital letters: "Benign Fibromuscular Stroma" was printed in black. The final tally: eleven out of the twelve samples were cancerous; each of them assigned a Gleason score of 8.

Reading this sobering report more than a year after being diagnosed, I fully understood that the high Gleason scores for eleven out of twelve cancerous cores meant that an aggressive cancer had overrun my prostate (and, as we shall see, had already migrated elsewhere). I was grateful I had not looked at the pathology report the day I learned of my diagnosis. The words, "You have a nasty prostate cancer," were scary enough on their own. There was no way I would have been mentally or emotionally prepared for this well-documented proof of what Dr. Hopkins had meant when he said that.

So, how did I end up with "high grade" prostate cancer? Answering this question required an exploration of my medical history.

MY GENITOURINARY HISTORY

Men have little reason to contemplate their prostate until something goes wrong with it. Unlike most of the male reproductive system, the prostate is tucked away into the lower pelvis, just underneath the bladder and against the wall of the rectum. A healthy prostate is about the size of a walnut, and its purpose is to secrete about one third of the seminal fluid that makes up the male ejaculate. Seminal fluid is vital to protect the ability of the sperm to survive and move (the technical term is "motility"). The prostate also contains some of the muscles that help expel semen during ejaculation.

The urethra, the tube leading from the bladder down through the penis, serves the dual purposes of ejaculation and urination; it is surrounded by the prostate gland just south of where the urethra exits the bladder. A normal prostate is important not only for the proper functioning of the male reproductive system, but to the health of the urinary tract as well.

As men are beginning to discover in increasing numbers, the prostate tends to swell as it ages, thereby constricting the urethra that passes through it. This swelling can lead to "male urinary symptoms," such as increased urinary frequency and the "weak stream" frequently highlighted in the numerous prescription drug ads seen on television. By and large, though, the entire male genitourinary system is an impressive and reliable piece of biological engineering.

Unfortunately, there are exceptions to this normally smooth functioning, and my genitourinary system had a history of malfunctions. I experienced my first urinary tract infection (UTI) in 1980. Men are rarely diagnosed with UTIs because the male urethra is a good deal longer than a woman's, and the bladder is reasonably distant from the wandering bacteria that can cause infections. That first UTI was sufficiently concerning that my primary care physician ordered a pyleogram, which X-rays both the kidneys and urinary tract. The same doctor also referred me to an urologist for a cystoscopy. Like the first fall off my bicycle as a young boy, I still have a clear memory of that first cysto. Upon encountering some sort of obstruction before arriving at the bladder itself, the urologist had pushed a bit harder on the flexible fiber optic snake making its way up my urethra. This was when the words "exquisite" and "pain" became immutably linked in my mind. At the conclusion of the exam, the doctor mentioned that the cystoscope appeared to have broken through some kind of urethral obstruction that may have caused the UTI. Finding nothing else out of the ordinary, however, he pronounced my urinary tract fit for service.

Which was mostly true, except that I continued to suffer periodically from UTIs at a rate of one about every two years or so. During subsequent appointments for these infections, doctors made dubiously insightful comments like, "Well, some men are more prone to UTIs than others. These antibiotics I'm prescribing will clear it up." The doctors were right: The antibiotics always seemed to do the trick—at least for a while.

In 2001, I was suffering from a particularly severe UTI, and my primary care physician referred me to Dr. Hopkins, the urologist who almost eight years later would diagnose my prostate cancer. Prior to our initial meeting, he ordered a complete blood panel, including a PSA test. This was the first time I'd undergone a blood test during a full-blown UTI. During my previous infections, the doctors had only taken urine samples to test for bacteria. The blood test revealed my PSA level was a worrisomely high 24 nanograms per milliliter (ng/ml). My first PSA test had occurred during a routine physical five years before when I turned fifty and at a level of about 1.5 had been pronounced "normal." This surge in PSA accompanying the UTI was when I first learned that other conditions besides prostate cancer can boost a man's PSA level.

During subsequent office visits over the next several weeks, Dr. Hopkins performed a variety of invasive tests, including rectal ultrasounds and a cystoscopy. As with my earlier UTIs, none of these procedures could identify a specific problem. Like all the doctors before him, he prescribed antibiotics, in this case a lengthy course of Cipro®, stating that the dosage should knock out the infection "once and for all." However, he remained concerned about my high PSA reading and scheduled a prostate biopsy. A prostate biopsy is among the most invasive of genitourinary tests, and I remember all the details of the two I have had. At the time of the first biopsy I worked in Boston and I recall Dr. Hopkins engaging me in casual conversation about the pennant outlook for the Boston Red Sox (this was 2001, so things didn't look good for the team), while he captured the 12 samples with his trusty spring-loaded instrument.

The biopsy revealed no cancerous cores, but it did result in an impressive multi-syllabic diagnosis—prostatic intraepithelial neoplasia (PIN), a benign condition of new cell formation in the prostate. Dr. Hopkins observed that there was some professional controversy about whether PIN eventually led to cancer, noting that approximately 30 to 40 percent of men with PIN were later diagnosed with prostate cancer. Ultimately, he identified the root cause of the high PSA score as an inflammation of the prostate ("prostatitis"), which normally healed on its own after a few weeks. However, he had no clue as to the root cause of my inflamed prostate other than to surmise it was bacterial in origin. A subsequent test about two months later showed that my PSA level had quieted back down to around 2.0, pleasing both of us. Dr. Hopkins and I then parted company, until seven years later, when I called for the appointment in late 2008. Since the 2001 PIN diagnosis I had no subsequent urinary tract infections, prostate symptoms, or abnormal PSA readings that would have motivated my primary care physician (or me) to call on Dr. Hopkins's services—or that of any other urologist—once again. During those seven years, all my genitourinary functions and metrics appeared to be "normal," including my PSA levels, with the one exception being the age-related swelling of my prostate—a.k.a. benign prostatic hyperplasia (BPH)—that was being treated by an alpha blocker drug to reduce the swelling and ease my ability to urinate. All seemed normal, even cured, since the UTIs had ceased—that is, until the mysterious blood that appeared in my urine in the fall of 2008.

ROOT CAUSES

Now that I had been diagnosed with prostate cancer, I wanted to know where it had come from. On the one hand, this information couldn't really help me since knowing the cancer's origin wouldn't influence how it would be treated. On the other hand, knowing the origins of my disease might help me absorb the emotional and psychological shock of my diagnosis. The orderly cause and effect world I preferred to inhabit did not easily accept the presence of cancer and the necessity of treatment. So, if cancer was the effect of something gone terribly wrong, I wondered what exactly that something might be.

First, there was my problematic genitourinary history. None of my male friends had experienced as many UTIs in their lives as I had, and none had undergone a prostate biopsy at the tender age of 54. (Or perhaps they had, but none of them had shared that personal information with me.) Did my medical history play a role in causing my prostate cancer? Perhaps. Or perhaps the UTIs, prostatitis, and the cancer were all somehow related and traced further back to some common origin. Or, maybe it was just the opposite: Perhaps they had little or nothing to do with each other.

Finding the root cause of any type of cancer is called etiology. Etiology requires an understanding of the mechanisms that create the DNA mutations (in most cancers) and gene fusions (in the case of prostate cancer) that transform healthy cells into cancerous ones. If researchers can figure out what causes the alterations in the cell's DNA, then they are on the way to understanding how to control those changes and ultimately to control— and perhaps even to cure—the disease itself.

It's difficult to overstate the complexity of the mechanisms of cell growth and the various signaling pathways that control both normal and abnormal (cancerous) growth. Scientists still have much to learn before they can achieve this elusive goal, although scores of researchers are working on this question. Cancer specialists have identified a host of genetic, environmental, and dietary risk factors that may increase the odds of many types of cancer, including prostate cancer. Risk factors associated with prostate cancer include, but are not limited to:

- age
- race
- family history
- consumption of dairy products, red meat, fats, and eggs
- excess testosterone
- sexually transmitted infections
- excess body weight
- smoking

Not every researcher agrees that all of these are definitive since there is no verifiable proof of a direct link between any particular risk factor and prostate cancer. As the authors of one prostate cancer study concluded, "Considerable work remains to further understand the etiology and translate the identification of risk factors into public recommendations and prevention strategies." Perhaps one or more of these possible causes had contributed to my present condition. There was also my history of prostatitis and the PIN. These factors seemed important, as least to my urologist. One day I asked Dr. Hopkins what he thought had caused my cancer. Without hesitation he replied, "Chronic prostatitis."

Chronic inflammation and infection are a known cause of other cancers, such as carcinomas of the stomach and liver. Researchers have been seeking evidence that an inflamed prostate (prostatitis) might lead to prostate cancer. One study of a database of prostate cancer patients found only a weak correlation, leading some medical experts to conclude, "These data do not provide compelling evidence for a role of chronic inflammation with prostate cancer." However, more recent research at the genetic level "suggest[s] that prostate cancer is associated with chronic inflammation," and "chronic inflammation may lead to cancer by a number of mechanisms." The next question is what mechanisms cause this kind of inflammation in the first place. Causes might include:

- bacteria
- viruses
- dietary habits (charred meat produces a well-known carcinogen)
- hormonal changes
- urine reflux
- physical trauma

Despite these possible causes, scientists argue,

Inflammation is a very complex process, which involves hundreds of genes ... that might contribute to the development of prostate cancer.

All we can conclude then, is that there is some evidence to suggest a link between inflammation and prostate cancer but any definitive link continues to elude scientists.

Given my history of UTIs and at least one known bout of prostatitis, Dr. Hopkins's hypothesis about the cause of my cancer seems correct. But of course the origins of my cancer—and doubtless all cancers—are like the layers of an onion: Peel away one cause, and the next one appears. The surest answer—although it feels like something of a cop out—is that it's a combination of factors. One thing I know for sure: I never smoked. All the other risk factors, in one way or another, remain on the table.

A BRIEF HISTORY OF PROSTATE CANCER

Cancer is an ancient disease. Egyptian hieroglyphs dating from 1500 BCE document breast cancer cases that were treated by cauterization. Hippocrates, and Galen after him, believed that an excess of black bile caused cancer, which was the dominant view of the disease until the 17th century. Not until the late 19th century did a theory emerge positing that cancerous cells were mutations of normal cells. A disease with the characteristics of prostate cancer was described as far back as the 16th century, but wasn't identified as a distinct disease until the middle of the 19th century.

A Prostate Cancer Timeline

1853 First case of prostate cancer reported

1904 First radical prostatectomy

1909 First radioactive implants

1937 National Cancer Institute (NCI) established

1941 Charles Huggins discovers testosterone deprivation slows prostate cancer growth

1966 Dr. Charles Gleason establishes a grading system to measure cancer aggressiveness

1971 Andrew Schally discovers the gonadotropin-releasing hormone (GnRH)

1979 Prostate specific androgen (PSA) isolated as a protein

1981 Widespread PSA testing initiated

1982 Dr. Patrick Walsh performs first nerve-sparing prostatectomy

1990 3D Conformal external beam radiotherapy (EBRT)

2010 Provenge®, first immunotherapy drug for any cancer, approved by FDA for use with prostate cancer

2011 United States Preventive Services Task Force (USPSTF) recommends against use of PSA test for community screening for prostate cancer

While all varieties of cancer are, at their essence, the same disease—cellular growth gone wild—each type of cancer has its own set of symptoms, a distinct spectrum of available treatments, and its own unique history. Although the prostate gland was first identified by the Venetian anatomist Niccolo Massa in 1536, the first case of prostate cancer was not officially reported in the medical literature until 1853, by J. Adams, a surgeon at the London Hospital. A 59-year-old man died from a prostate tumor that had spread to his lymph nodes three years after the onset of his symptoms. Dr. Adams claimed that the condition was "a very rare disease." Because of the shorter life expectancies and poor detection techniques of the time, doctors continued to believe the condition was rare until well into the beginning of the twentieth century.

The earliest documented treatment for prostate cancer involved surgeries to remove urinary obstructions. In the late 1890s, orchiectomy (the surgical removal of the testicles, i.e., castration) was tried on several patients, with limited success. Dr. Hugh Young first removed the entire prostate gland (radical perineal prostatectomy) at Johns Hopkins Hospital in 1904. At first, the prostate removal surgery was intended to alleviate symptoms, but it soon became the preferred treatment for a possible cure. But the price paid by the patient was high: a complete inability to have erections and the possibility for permanent incontinence. So doctors continued to pursue alternative therapies.

In 1895, Wilhelm Roentgen discovered the X-ray. He and other researchers soon realized that X-rays damaged cancerous cells more than healthy ones, and that healthy cells could recover and continue to form new cells, while cancer cells could not. By the early twentieth century, radiation therapy (or radiotherapy) had become an important tool in the treatment of many different cancers. The potential for radiation to help cancer patients increased when Marie Curie isolated the radioactive elements of radium and polonium as part of her doctoral research in 1903. In 1909, radioactive implants—a precursor of today's brachytherapy— began to be used to treat prostate cancer as a regular course of treatment.

By the eve of World War II, prostate cancer—and cancer in general—was no longer viewed as a "rare" disease. In 1900, cancer was the ninth leading cause of death in America; by the 1930s, it was second only to heart disease. Because many cancers occur later in life, cancer's increased prevalence was in part due to the longer life expectancies of the general population. In 1937, the government created the National Cancer Institute to increase funding and support for research into the disease. In the fourteen years that followed, funding for cancer research increased twenty-fold, reaching more than 14 million dollars annually by 1951. In recent years, the U.S. government has spent about 5.5 billion dollars annually for cancer research. Cancer rose ever higher in the nation's consciousness during the middle of the twentieth century, and the disease has remained one of America's top health concerns ever since, leading to President Richard Nixon's declaration of a "war on cancer" in the early 1970s.

Since 1893, when the surgeon W.J. White published a paper on the effects of castration on the size of the prostate in dogs, doctors had known that there was some link between testosterone and the growth of prostate cancer. Although orchiectomies were occasionally performed, the debilitating side effects of the surgery were not usually worth the potential gains. A major breakthrough in hormone treatment came from Charles B. Huggins, a Canadian scientist, in 1941. Huggins discovered that the female hormone, estrogen, could be used to counteract the effects of testosterone in men, including testosterone's ability to stimulate prostate cancer growth. In 1966, Huggins won the Nobel Prize for his discovery.

This was the first time hormones were used to control the growth of a cancer, and in the mid-1940s, estrogen therapy, called "hormone ablation," began to eclipse radiation as the preferred treatment for prostate cancer. Because detection methods were more primitive than those of today, prostate cancer was typically not caught until it had spread (metastasized), usually to the patient's bones. Hormone ablation was a helpful treatment innovation because it proved effective against advanced prostate cancer that had already metastasized, significantly extending patients' survival, sometimes by years.

Radiotherapy regained some of its former popularity in the 1950s, as more powerful X-ray technologies—notably the linear accelerator—allowed for the development of external beam radiation therapy (EBRT). The first patients treated with EBRT had inoperable tumors, and by the late 1950s, researcher Malcolm Bagshaw and others were reporting that radiation alone had the potential to cure prostate cancer. Over the next two decades, higher-energy accelerators and three-dimensional imaging enabled the prostate to be treated more precisely with increasingly higher doses of radiation, while also sparing more of the surrounding healthy tissue. In the 1960s, doctors began to experiment with combining hormone ablation and radiation therapy. They found that, in certain cases, giving hormone treatment in advance of EBRT would shrink the prostate to a more favorable size and shape for radiation. This combination therapy is still used, especially for inoperable tumors, albeit using today's more sophisticated drugs and radiotherapy technologies. As it turned out, this treatment course ended up to be the best one for me.

A significant advance in prostate cancer diagnosis came in 1966, when Dr. Donald Gleason developed the Gleason score, a grading system to measure the aggressiveness of prostate tumors. Prior to the Gleason score, there was no single system to describe the relative aggressiveness of the different cellular forms of prostate cancer. Dr. Gleason's technique, which he first published in *Cancer Chemotherapy Reports* in 1966, focused on the architecture of the cancer cells. He rated the appearance of the cells and assigned each sample a grade ranging from 1 to 5, with 1 being a normal, healthy cell, and 5 being the most cancerous looking, a malformed, "undifferentiated" shape and consistency that barely looked like a cell at all. He assigned a grade of 1 to 5 to the most frequently occurring patterns of cells found in the tumor, and then a second grade between 1 and 5 to the next most predominant pattern of cells. Adding the two grades together gave the Gleason score (GS)—ranging from 2 (1 + 1) to 10 (5 + 5)—to the tumor. In general, the lower the Gleason score at the time of diagnosis, the less aggressive the cancer and the more favorable the patient's prognosis.

In 1971, Andrew Schally discovered the gonadotropin-releasing hormone (GnRH)—also known by the equally unwieldy term, luteinizing hormone-releasing hormone (LHRH). Injecting the patient with an "LHRH agonist" mimics the action of the naturally occurring hormone, effectively tricking the brain into thinking sufficient testosterone has been produced in the testicles, causing them to shut off further production of the male hormone. In 1977, Drs. Schally and Guillemin won the Nobel Prize for their work in GnRH synthesis, which led to the creation of a class of drugs known as testosterone inactivating pharmaceuticals (TIP) used for androgen ablation (otherwise known as androgen suppression, androgen deprivation therapy [ADT], or more forthrightly, chemical castration—all lumped under the euphemistic rubric, "hormone therapy"). These drugs came to replace estrogen as the hormone treatment for prostate cancer, a distinct advantage because these new drugs avoided estrogen's potential for causing lethal heart problems. Later, anti-androgen drugs were developed that could specifically block the testosterone receptors (also called androgen receptors) in both normal cells and cancer cells. Anti-androgens could be used alone or in conjunction with ADT to prevent testosterone from feeding the growth of the cancer cells.

In 1979, a team of researchers isolated prostate-specific antigen (PSA), a protein that is generated exclusively by both healthy and cancerous prostate cells, leading to the development of the PSA blood test in 1980. It was only after the growing use of the PSA test began to substantially increase the number of prostate cancers being diagnosed in their earlier stages that the Gleason score became widely used. In 1987, seven urology experts recommended its uniform use in all scientific publications in order to encourage greater uniformity in evaluating tumors.

But while an elevated PSA can suggest the possibility of cancer in the prostate, it is far from a definitive test for cancer. Ideally, the first PSA test occurs for a man at around age 50 (or earlier if he has a family history of prostate cancer or is African American). This first test establishes a "baseline" value. If a subsequent test shows an increase in the PSA level, a digital rectal exam (DRE) performed by an experienced doctor can help indicate whether a tumor might be present. Generally, only a suspicious DRE, together with a PSA value that has increased from an earlier test, should lead to a prostate biopsy.

PSA levels are affected by other factors besides prostate cancer. As I had found out in 2001 when prostatitis had elevated my PSA level, PSA concentration in the blood will rise due to a variety of causes, including sexual activity and UTIs, as well as prostate cancer. An increasing PSA level is the critical issue, but even then a higher score does not necessarily mean that something proportionately worse is happening. And, as I knew from personal experience, cancer can occur with a seemingly "normal" PSA value. While my PSA had risen to 24 ng/ml during my 2001 bout with prostatitis, my Gleason 8 aggressive cancer had not even budged my PSA level above 1.5, substantially less than the generally accepted "normal" limit of 4 ng/ml (or even above more recent guidelines that suggest any PSA greater than 2.0 in men 55 or older deserves follow up). In sum, PSA is an indicator of possible cancer, but it is an unreliable one—and it says absolutely nothing about the cancer's aggressiveness. That's why a prostate biopsy is always necessary to confirm or deny cancer's existence and, if it's present, to measure its extent and aggressiveness. Nevertheless, the PSA test remains the most widely used, although controversial, means of early prostate cancer detection.

The effect of the PSA test on the number of prostate cancers diagnosed has been enormous; in 1980, about 85 thousand cases were diagnosed; by 1990, there were about 200 thousand new cases reported. Since 1990, the number of newly diagnosed prostate cancer cases has remained between 175 thousand and 225 thousand each year in the United States. This has led some to question the widespread use of the PSA test because of concerns that high PSA readings tend to lead to over-diagnosis of prostate cancer.

Results published in 2009 from two ongoing studies in the US and Europe suggested that widespread PSA screening has not provided a net benefit in reducing prostate cancer mortality rates. These studies have proved controversial since they are based on only ten years of data—an insufficient amount of time to reach a definitive conclusion, at least in the opinion of many. In addition, many researchers and doctors have questioned the methodology of the studies themselves. In 2011, the United States Preventive Services Task Force (USPSTF) appeared to rely heavily on these study data when the panel issued a recommendation that "community wide" PSA screening of healthy males be discontinued, or at least discouraged. Not surprisingly, a public outcry ensued—similar in intensity to the outcry a few years earlier when the same panel made its recommendation to discourage use of mammograms to screen healthy women for breast cancer. While the USPSTF recommendation doubtless made sense at a statistical level, the many men who asserted that without a PSA test their cancer would have metastasized and killed them highlighted the reality that in the end, disease is more than statistics: It is about individual lives.

The underlying problem lies in the nature of the cancer itself. Approximately 80 percent of diagnosed prostate tumors are classified as "indolent" or slow growing, while the other 20 percent are aggressive. Given its generally slow-growing nature and therefore the reduced probability of the cancer ever causing actual harm, prostate cancer can be over-treated, where the "Cure is worse than the disease," leading too often to incontinence and impotence—complications that could have been avoided by choosing to forego surgery or radiation altogether. Some slow-growing prostate cancers in older men, for example, may not need to be treated at all, although choosing to do nothing—known as "expectant management" or "active surveillance"—can be a difficult psychological decision for a man to make. Current research is directed at finding a more definitive and accurate blood test: one that would use genetic markers ("biomarkers") to differentiate clearly between relatively slow-growing tumors and aggressive forms of this cancer. This will not be an easy task since among other complexities, more than twenty-seven genetic variants of prostate cancer have been indentified so far.

PSA has one other important and reasonably uncontroversial use. It is the metric by which the state of post-treatment health of prostate cancer survivors is judged. In almost all cases, prostate cancer cells are enthusiastic emitters of PSA. As long as the PSA level remains low (preferably undetectable) and steady, then the cancer is deemed to not have returned in strength. But if PSA levels begin to rise after surgery, radiation, or hormone treatment, then the cancer is assumed to have returned and further treatment will be called for.

With increasing numbers of prostate cancer diagnoses, advances continued to be made in the three major treatments for the disease: hormone ablation, surgery, and radiation. In 1982, Dr. Patrick Walsh performed the first "nerve-sparing" prostatectomy, which could help preserve sexual and urinary function following surgery. In 1992, laparoscopic radical prostatectomy was introduced for early stage "localized" cancers that are still wholly contained within the prostate gland. Today, robotic-assisted laparoscopic surgery has become an increasingly popular method for removing localized cancers. However, as we will see, there's still substantial controversy about the relative advantages of each kind of surgery.

Brachytherapy—the implantation of radioactive seeds in the prostate—was developed to treat localized prostate cancers in 1983. By 1990, 3D conformal external beam radiotherapy began to be used as a treatment for more advanced cases of prostate cancer. Intensity-modulated radiotherapy (IMRT) and more recently, subsets of IMRT, such as image-guided radiotherapy (IGRT) and tomotherapy, which image the location of the prostate before commencing that day's therapy, have provided the ability to focus radiation even more precisely on the prostate, avoiding damage to surrounding tissues and reducing the urinary and bowel side effects that often accompany traditional radiotherapy. A competing form of radiation technology is proton beam radiotherapy (PBRT), which uses high-energy protons instead of photons (X-rays) as its radiation source. This technology provides extreme accuracy with virtually no stray radiation to damage surrounding tissue. However, PBRT is controversial because of its high cost and the absence of studies definitively demonstrating its superiority over less expensive and increasingly accurate IMRT technologies.

Most prostate cancer patients initially respond well to some combination of surgery, radiation (IMRT, PBRT, and/or brachytherapy), and hormone therapy. Over time, however, men with more aggressive tumors (typically, Gleason 8 or greater) are likely to develop androgen-independent (called "hormone-refractory" or "castrate resistant") cancer that ceases to respond to hormone therapy. This has led some researchers to study the effectiveness of chemotherapy in late-stage prostate cancer. Early studies in the 1960s and 1970s found that chemotherapy was only minimally effective in treating these cancers (measured by the relative decrease in PSA level). More recent studies with newer chemotherapy drugs such as docetaxel have shown significant improvement, however, with 50 to 75 percent of men exhibiting a decrease in PSA after chemotherapy.

Other types of treatment for prostate cancer remain in their experimental stages. Some surgeons now offer cryosurgery, a technique that alternately freezes and thaws the prostate tissue, ultimately destroying it, but it is unclear whether cryosurgery is as effective as traditional surgery. There is also high frequency ultrasound (HIFU), which uses radio frequencies to rapidly heat the prostate, destroying both healthy and cancerous cells in the process. As of this writing, neither cryotherapy nor HIFU has been approved by the FDA for use in the United States. As well, there is a variety of alternative medicine therapies, most involving herbs. These therapies have had salutary effects for some individuals. The Memorial Sloan-Kettering website lists hundreds of herbs used to treat cancer—although they are unproven, and the FDA officially sanctions none of them.

Some experiments and clinical trials are underway to study immunological treatments, including a variety of vaccines and antibodies. One such drug, Provenge®, was approved by the FDA in 2010, and is the first treatment for any type of cancer that harnesses the body's own immune system to attack cancerous cells and reduce their proliferation. The goal of these treatments is to treat advanced prostate cancer patients who are castrate resistant without the potentially dangerous side effects of chemotherapy.

Because prostate cancer affects so many men, doctors, researchers, and pharmaceutical companies will continue to work to improve detection accuracy and treatment. In economic terms, prostate cancer treatment represents a large market opportunity—and every man diagnosed with this disease will hopefully benefit from this reality. But that is a discussion for later. My personal encounter with the world of prostate cancer treatment was only just beginning.

THREE

Boarding the Oncology Adventure Ride

DIAGNOSTIC CODE 185

When I was a kid, my favorite ride at Disneyland was Space Mountain, a high-speed rollercoaster housed inside an enormous windowless room. With its sudden drops and sharp turns, Space Mountain was far more exciting than an ordinary roller coaster because the all-encompassing darkness prevented me from seeing what was coming next. A roller coaster in a dark room is an apt metaphor for cancer diagnosis and treatment—what I came to call the Oncology Adventure Ride. As with Space Mountain on a busy summer day, the rider, or in this case, the cancer patient, must be prepared to wait in line for the adventure to begin. Just as on a roller coaster, it is the system's managers—not you—that determine the speed of progress from initial diagnosis through additional testing to actual treatment. And once you board the ride, you can control little more than how nervously you shift in your seat. The Oncology Adventure Ride moves on tracks, following a predetermined course, and it is basically impossible to get off until the end of the ride. As with Space Mountain, there are always surprises in store. A gradual ascent to the top of the ride may lull you into thinking that you know exactly what is going to happen next. Suddenly, there is a dramatic downhill acceleration and an unexpectedly sharp 90-degree turn. Slow ascents alternate with hair-raising descents. Finally, at the end of the ride, you exit, disoriented, a bit worse for wear. Something about you is different, but you are not quite sure yet what it is.

"You have a nasty prostate cancer." The words were real enough, but their meaning had not yet penetrated the mental fog that had descended on me that January morning at Pacific Urology. "Actually you have an aggressive cancer, Gleason eight," Dr. Hopkins continued. My brain gradually absorbed the implication of the adjective "aggressive" modifying the noun "cancer." My mental fog was not so thick that I didn't realize this diagnosis was serious business.

Sitting on the patient's side of Dr.Hopkins's desk, I managed to organize enough brain cells to ask feebly, "So, what does Gleason eight mean?"

"The Gleason scoring system is how the pathologist assesses the prostate biopsy samples," Dr. Hopkins explained. "Cancerous cells are more irregular in shape and size than healthy ones. The more irregular the cell pattern—we call it 'undifferentiated'—the higher the Gleason score, which tops out at ten. Your score of eight means that your cancer is aggressive and growing quickly."

The office suddenly felt colder. I became aware of my heart beating quickly and my breath becoming shallow. Somewhere deep inside me, my primitive brain was signaling my body to prepare for the next piece of not-so-great news.

If Dr. Hopkins noticed the pallor in my face, he didn't mention it, but continued efficiently dispensing the relevant medical information. "The first thing we need to do is halt the cancer's growth. Prostate cancer feeds off testosterone, so we need to cut off its food supply. There are two ways to do this. The first is called androgen deprivation therapy, ADT for short. It almost completely shuts down testosterone production in your body. ADT comes with significant side effects, including muscle mass loss, osteoporosis, and weight gain."

A few days later, while doing my own research, I discovered a much longer list of unpleasant side effects created by ADT.

Other consequences of turning off testosterone production include gynecomastia (breast growth), anemia, fatigue, decreases in HDL ("good cholesterol"), and depression. And of course the biggest—but perhaps the least surprising—effect is the complete loss of sexual function, which is at least tempered by an accompanying loss of libido.

"So, given the downsides of ADT," Dr. Hopkins continued, "I would prefer to use a more cutting-edge therapy without as many side effects. It's widely used in Europe but is not as popular here in the United States."

"I'm all for cutting-edge," I said.

"Good," Dr. Hopkins replied. "We'll use an anti-androgen drug called Casodex®, also called bicalutamide. It doesn't stop testosterone production. Instead, it prohibits your testosterone from attaching to a part of the prostate cell called an androgen receptor, including the androgen receptors of the cancerous cells. This should slow the growth of the cancer, as well as shrink the size of your prostate, which will make it easier to treat. Recent research says that the relatively high dose I'm going to prescribe is as effective as ADT in halting your cancer's growth, but without all the side effects."

To a mind completely uneducated about prostate cancer, much less its treatment, all that sounded good, but I suspected that there would be some drawbacks. "So, what are the downsides of the anti-androgen?" I asked.

Dr. Hopkins explained, "The most significant side effect is breast enlargement with tenderness. To counteract that, I'll prescribe a drug, tamoxifen, which is used to treat women with breast cancer. That should help reduce the swelling."

His explanation was interrupted by a phone call. Hearing only Dr. Hopkins's side of the conversation, I deduced that it was one of his colleagues calling from an operating room. The caller was apparently seeking some surgical advice. Dr. Hopkins responded with a few anatomically technical suggestions and wished the caller good luck.

Given my distressed state, this was a reassuring interruption. Not only did it give me a chance to take a deep breath, but it provided important information, as well. The fact that other surgeons called Dr. Hopkins for guidance meant that they valued his expertise. As his patient, this was comforting. With all the bad news that I had just heard, I was ready to feel reassured by anything I could hold onto.

We ended our conversation at the appointment desk as he filled out my prescription and lab test forms. "We also need to schedule a urethral biopsy to follow up on that lesion I saw during the cystoscopy," Dr. Hopkins said. Then he changed the subject and stated disconcertingly, "you know, you really should have been seeing me every six months since we diagnosed the PIN eight years ago. I would have caught this sooner."

Great, I thought. Not only do I have cancer, as well as some kind of lesion in my urethra, but now he tells me, "if only." Having no idea what to make of his assertion, I replied the same way I did when I found out our company had lost an important order, "Well, we are where we are. Unfortunately, it's water under the bridge."

Later, as I reflected on the "if only," I was not so much regretful as angry. I was angry at the medical insurance system that had planted my primary care physician firmly in the way as a gatekeeper, blocking access to the urologist. (I have since obtained a more expensive form of health insurance that allows me to see specialists directly.) I was also annoyed at Dr. Hopkins for pointing out a fact that could no longer be changed. Above all, I was mad at myself for not following up more diligently on the prostatic interepithelial neoplasia (PIN) diagnosed in 2001 that had apparently evolved into actual prostate cancer sometime during 2008. Why, I pondered, was I able to think strategically when it came to marketing electronic equipment, but was completely clueless when it came to thinking strategically about my own health?

Dr. Hopkins interrupted my self-critical reflection and announced, "We'll meet for a pre-surgical consultation before the urethral biopsy. See you then." At the bottom of one of the forms was a spaced marked "diagnosis, primary." To the right of these words Dr. Hopkins had scrawled the number "185."

I walked out of the Pacific Urology office feeling far more disoriented than when I had walked in. My surroundings were identical, the weather unchanged, but I was not the same man who had entered the building just two hours earlier. I had undergone a metamorphosis: I was now a cancer patient—a whole different type of person, someone I never imagined that I would become. Before this moment, I had let myself believe that cancer only happened to other people.

A few minutes later, Susan came to pick me up in the parking lot. After I climbed wordlessly into the passenger seat and shut the door, she began driving to the exit. Suddenly, without looking at her, I blurted out, "I have prostate cancer." She slammed on the brakes and pulled over. Turning and staring wide-eyed, she uttered a quiet and disbelieving, "What?" The shocked look on her face was the perfect illustration of what I felt, now that the gray mist of incomprehension was beginning to evaporate.

I repeated the four words slowly and distinctly as much to myself as to Susan, "I have prostate cancer."

Almost immediately I kicked myself, realizing that this was about the most insensitive way possible to convey the bad news. Why couldn't I have taken a more humane approach, and at least prepared her by saying something like, "I love you, and I'm afraid I have some bad news"? But it was too late for sensitivity now. At the moment I laid eyes on the person I loved the most, I could say nothing other than to repeat the same scary words that I had just heard in the doctor's office. In my shock, these words were all that mattered, and they seemed to have fallen out of my mouth on their own.

Slowly, both of us began to find our words. "I'm so sorry," I said. "I should have prepared you first."

"You're right, but this is shocking news," she responded. "What happens now?" She put the car in gear and continued driving as our conversation veered away from the emotional shock. Instinctively, we both sought neutral territory and began to discuss some of the medical logistics that would soon be consuming much of our lives.

GLOOMY REFLECTIONS

I am sure that everyone who receives a cancer diagnosis feels something different when they first hear the news—perhaps terror, anger, disbelief, denial, or even sadness might be the first emotion to arise. My initial feeling upon hearing Dr. Hopkins's pronouncement was a strange detachment. Looking back, I realize that this feeling of disconnection was shock, the same shock that led me to blurt out my news so suddenly to Susan. Once my brain was able to process the information, however, I felt within myself a call to action. I had just been thrust into the world of cancer, about which I was completely ignorant. My first, most powerful instinct was to find out as much as possible about cancer in general and prostate cancer in particular. I felt that I needed to understand more—and fast—starting with that mysterious "185" that Dr. Hopkins had written in the primary diagnosis box on the lab order he handed me.

I already knew that the numbers doctors write on their forms are part of a standardized diagnostic coding system. Later that day, I entered "diagnostic codes" into Google's search box and discovered that there is a worldwide coding system developed by the World Health Organization called the International Classification of Diseases, or ICD9. Staring back at me from the computer screen, the definition for diagnostic code 185 was *malignant neoplasm of the prostate*—prostate cancer in everyday language or the abbreviated PCa (or occasionally, CaP) in professional jargon. I had just joined the approximately 200,000 men in the United States who have "185" written into their medical records each year.

Cancer is a simple two-syllable word with immense life-changing power. Up to this point, whenever I heard someone's name in the same sentence as cancer, I thought, "Oh, wow, that's really awful for them." But since it was about someone else, cancer remained a safe abstraction. After all, it was their disease, not mine. But not anymore. Now cancer was mine. What had always been an intangible condition had suddenly become a concrete reality. I felt a strange combination of confusion and disbelief. Like the near-death experiences people sometimes describe, I felt as though I had stepped outside of myself and was watching from somewhere high above, thinking, "Who is he? Oh he's the guy with cancer."

My mind started to wander into irrational territory. This diagnosis must be a mistake, an administrative error of some kind, I thought. During an initial moment of disbelief, I was positive that Dr. Hopkins had been handed the wrong pathology report, and that it actually belonged to someone else. Over the next few days, I began to wake up in the morning to find myself playing a new game: How many minutes (seconds?)

would pass before I would remember that I, Craig Pynn, had prostate cancer?

It is difficult to imagine a disease more ingeniously designed to attack manhood at its core. But it was much more than my sexual identity that was threatened. I was also plunged unwillingly into the subservient role of patient, an unnatural state for someone who was used to taking charge and getting things done. In 1995, I had been involved in a car accident that led to a seven-day hospital stay. As I healed, I grew bored and wanted nothing more than to be released and reenter the world that did not categorize me—and treat me—as the submissive "patient." This time, I wasn't going to be confined to the hospital—at least not yet—but I was going to have to be a "patient" for much longer than seven days. Worse, I was now a *cancer patient*, and God only knew what invasive, possibly painful, procedures lay in store.

A cancer diagnosis initially leads to mostly self-centered thoughts, but I now began to wonder: What about my family? Cancer certainly puts to the test the "in sickness and in health" section of my marriage vows to my wife, Susan, spoken forty years earlier. She already had secondary progressive multiple sclerosis. Now I had cancer. We were now both living with serious diseases. My thoughts and emotions were taking me down some dark paths: "How much time do I really have? What about our children and grandchildren? What about our retirement plans? What if...?"

OVERCOMING IGNORANCE

Waiting to board a roller coaster can be a mix of trepidation and excitement. Although they may be nervous, prospective riders have plenty of evidence to suggest that they will survive. This helps minimize their fear. The Oncology Adventure Ride works much the same way. For data-driven people like me, understanding the details of prostate cancer, its diagnosis, its treatment, and its likely course helps to manage the anxiety that naturally accompanies the disease.

First, I wanted to know how I ended up waiting to board the Oncology Adventure Ride in the first place. I had been diligent about having annual physicals with my primary care physician. And each of these check-ups always included a digital rectal exam (DRE). My prostate-specific antigen (PSA) level had been rock-steady at less than 2.0 nanograms per milliliter (ng/ml) ever since my last visit with Dr. Hopkins almost eight years previously. My most recent PSA was 1.53, taken just seven months ago. I had read somewhere that a PSA reading less than 4.0 ng/ml was considered "normal." Like many other men, I believed that a normal PSA level meant a healthy prostate. So, how could I have a low PSA reading and a nasty cancer simultaneously? Apparently, the relationship between PSA and cancer was not quite as simple as I had first believed.

Also, Dr. Hopkins said I had aggressive cancer, and we needed to stop its growth quickly. He also said the conventional ADT treatment had a lot of downsides. But his prescription for a high dose of an anti-androgen drug had not been used widely in the United States. Why not? Maybe I should seek a second opinion from another doctor. But I didn't even know how to frame my question yet. I needed to do some preliminary research first.

Prior to the twenty-first century, researching diseases was an arduous task, involving trips to well-stocked research libraries. The only other reliable option was to seek second opinions from other experts in the field. With the advent of the Internet, self-diagnosis became the new rage. Medical assistants at numerous doctors' offices are now required to field phone calls from hysterical patients who have Googled their symptoms and diagnosed themselves with a terminal illness based only on vague information. As a result, medical staffs must now spend valuable time convincing these people that the doctor's diagnosis and treatment recommendations are in fact correct.

The Internet is a useful tool, which like other sharp-edged tools needs to be used with care. It augments, but does not replace, sound medical opinion from an experienced practitioner who has examined both the data and the body in question. While I knew the dangers of self-diagnosis based on information found online, I still wanted to take advantage of the wide availability of medical data to reassure myself that Dr. Hopkins's treatment recommendations were truly my best options. But, at this point, prostate cancer was still basically a mystery to me. Not only did I lack the knowledge to understand what treatment strategies might be the best ones, but it was also still way too early to start weighing the pros and cons of treatment alternatives. I still had many diagnostic tests to undergo—including the ominous-sounding urethral biopsy. I felt incompetent to make any kind of rational decision about choosing between two different types of drugs to treat a disease about which I knew essentially nothing.

"Would you prefer the anti-androgen drug or ADT?" This was doubtless just the first of many decisions that I would make—or appear to make—many of which could have life-altering consequences. Was choosing the anti-androgen drug instead of ADT a good decision or not? How could I know? How many other decisions was I about to make—or worse, how many other decisions might be made for me—that would be less than ideal? The feeling of helplessness was overwhelming. What had become of the Craig Pynn I thought I was, the rational engineer and businessperson who considered decisions strategically? He now felt like nothing more than a clueless patient wandering lost in a dangerous medical wilderness.

Of course, I knew I should trust the doctor's professional judgment and experience, which I suppose I did. I was certainly not the first man to be diagnosed with prostate cancer. If you have to get cancer, it is probably better to get a relatively common one. Prostate cancer has seen intensive research, thousands of clinical studies, and a surfeit of curative therapies. I remembered reading that almost everyone who gets prostate cancer now survives it. This was reassuring information, but as I processed my own diagnosis, my unspoken fear was that I would be one of the exceptions.

So where should I start? All cancer patients develop important relationships with their doctors. Some patients choose to trust and accept their doctors' advice without question, trusting the medical system to do the right thing for them. But others, like me, want to gather our own information, weighing our doctors' advice against the other opinions that are out there. By making the effort to read the medical myself, I could take comfort knowing that my doctor's diagnosis and treatment recommendations were supported by reliable data. And if what the doctor tells me sounds contrary to what I have learned on my own, I will be far better prepared to ask questions in greater depth. Above all, I want to participate in the decision-making process without feeling that the important choices had been made without my input.

PROSTATE CANCER 101

When first diagnosed, I knew virtually nothing about prostate cancer. I only knew it was a "prostate," not a "prostrate," as I had heard many men mispronounce it. I had no idea what a Gleason score was. The terms "anti-androgen" and "androgen deprivation therapy" were completely foreign. I did not even know that prostate cancer grows by feeding off a man's testosterone. The only thing I knew about my prostate was that it was enlarged, and I had been taking an alpha-blocker drug for the past eight years to make it easier to urinate. Clearly, I had much to learn.

The education of Craig Pynn, uninformed cancer patient, began by typing "prostate cancer" into Google. This proved a bit overwhelming when the search returned more than twelve million web pages that mentioned the words "prostate" or "cancer." Next, I tried Amazon.com, typing in "prostate cancer book," the results of which were almost twelve hundred books and articles related to prostate cancer. The majority of these titles dealt with clinical issues, ranging from medical textbooks to *Prostate Cancer for Dummies* to specialized topics such as *The Prostate Cancer Diet*. There were numerous books whose agendas were clear from their titles, such as *The Natural Prostate Cure*, *Surviving Prostate Cancer without Surgery*, or *The Prostate Miracle: New Natural Therapies*. Many books argued for the superiority of certain treatment options, from proton beam therapy to robotic surgery to natural cures, such as saw palmetto leaves or pomegranate juice. While there was a surfeit of recommendations, there was a comparable lack of books written in the first person that delivered straightforward information describing the experiences and feelings of real men who had been diagnosed and treated for prostate cancer.

I had to narrow my search to find the information that could help me. But how? What did I really need to know? It was obviously too late to bother with information about which diet or what herbs would help me avoid prostate cancer. Likewise, it was really still too early to think about treatment options, although that would come soon enough. Eventually, I decided that the nature, diagnosis, and classification of prostate cancer as a disease were the first things that I needed to understand.

On the day Dr. Hopkins wrote "185" on my lab form, there were two things about prostate cancer that I wanted to know right away. First, what was it about my Gleason score that caused him to say, "You have a nasty cancer?" This hardly seemed like the kind of reassurance a doctor would want to give to a newly diagnosed patient. Second, what were the experiences of other men who possessed the same "nasty cancer" as I? As I learned more over the next few weeks, these two questions formed the basis of what I came to think of as the "two tracks of learning about prostate cancer." First, there is the scientific "fact track." Second, there is the more personal "experience track" that describes a man's physical and emotional encounter with prostate cancer. The personal experiences of other men like me were really what I was more curious about. But initially, facts proved easier to find. Facts like one in six American men will be diagnosed with prostate cancer. Also, if autopsies were to be performed on the other five after they had died of other causes, cancerous prostate cells would be found in most of them. These men just never knew they had cancer. About 80 percent of prostate cancers are slow growing, "indolent" in the professional jargon, and never announce themselves with a symptom beyond a slowly rising PSA. But the other 20 percent are fast growing and aggressive. These are the forms of prostate cancer most likely to result in rapidly rising PSAs or worse, symptoms such as the urinary bleeding that I had experienced. These are the cancers with high Gleason scores.

Googling "Gleason score" narrowed the search results to a mere two hundred fifteen thousand pages. Entering "Gleason score 8" halved that number to one hundred twenty-six thousand. This was where Google's proprietary algorithms that rank relevant pages proved useful. The summaries of the highly ranked pages contained the abstracts that looked the most promising.

When researching a disease like prostate cancer, one needs to be prepared to read some not-so-reassuring (maybe even frightening) information without jumping to unsound conclusions. Google's highest ranked page was www.prostate-cancer.org, which featured a scientific paper entitled, "The Gleason Score: A Significant Biologic Manifestation of Prostate Cancer Aggressiveness on Biopsy." The paper stated that of a sample of fifty-four thousand prostate cancer cases between 1994 and 1998, only

17 percent had Gleason scores between eight and ten. I was not so sure that I liked this kind of exclusivity. Perhaps it was Google's virtual humor at work, but the second most highly ranked page in my search was www.dummies.com, which stated simply and without elaboration, "Gleason scores from eight to ten indicate that the cancer is highly aggressive."

"Uh, oh," I thought. "This doesn't look good." But I didn't want to get ahead of myself. There were other facts to consider, like my low PSA of 1.5 when I was diagnosed. Perhaps this low reading would offset some of the bad news about the Gleason score. All of the articles I'd read so far talked about high PSA readings correlating to cancer. So, what was the deal with a score that was within the normal range? "How can I have a low PSA and an aggressive cancer at the same time?" I wondered.

At that moment, I realized I had just formulated the first question to ask Dr. Hopkins at our next meeting. My final act during this on-line session on the Internet was to order a copy of *Prostate Cancer for Dummies*. I needed an overview of the entire disease, and there was no question at this point that the publishers of that popular series of books had used a title that fitted me perfectly.

Some Websites for Learning About Prostate Cancer

The "Fact Track":

National Cancer Institute (cancer.gov/prostate)

American Cancer Society (cancer.org)

Prostate Cancer Research Institute (prostate-cancer.org)

Prostate Cancer Foundation (pcf.org)

The "Experience Track":

Cancer Survivors Network, American Cancer Society (csn.cancer.org)

Malecare: Men Fighting Cancer, Together (malecare.org)

The New Prostate Cancer InfoLink Social Network (prostatecancerinfolink.ning.com)

Us TOO International (www.ustoo.org)

You Are Not Alone Now Prostate Cancer Support Site (www.yananow.org)

A few days later, I was back at the computer looking for information on the "Experience Track." I had recently signed up for an account on Facebook in order to see what my adult children were doing. Maybe there was some kind of social networking site for prostate cancer. I typed "prostate cancer social network" into Google, and a link to "The 'New' Prostate Cancer InfoLink Social Network" appeared at the top of the results page. This discovery led to many hours of reading about other men's experiences with prostate cancer, and even a few stories of men with aggressive forms like mine. Since then, I've discovered other sites, such as the Cancer Survivors Network, sponsored by the American Cancer Society, another sponsored by Us TOO International, a prostate cancer advocacy organization, Malecare, another advocacy group, and YANA Now, a site featuring prostate cancer experiences written by men from around the world. These websites reflected men's honest stories, frank questions, and genuine worries. Just knowing that there were other men out there in similar circumstances helped to take the foreboding clinical edge off what I had learned earlier on the "fact track." These were stories of men afflicted with prostate cancer, but most of them were still living productive lives. Some of the experiences they described were frightening; others were more encouraging. But each story I read revealed an undercurrent of grit, tenacity, and a fervent drive to get both their minds and hearts around what was happening to them. Clearly, men were getting through this, even though it was a challenging journey. I felt better, but I was not ready to join any social networks just yet. My story was still too new and undeveloped, my feelings still too raw, and my thoughts too incoherent to begin to share them with others.

At least now I was a bit more informed on the fact side, and somewhat more encouraged on the experience side. Above all, I felt better prepared for my next meeting with Dr. Hopkins. Metaphorically, I was still standing at the front of the line, getting ready to board the Oncology Adventure Ride, with a little—just a little—less trepidation. The cars were pulling into the platform in front of me; I could see my seat. I was ready to climb aboard. What I did not know yet was that the ride would start right off with a sharp, unexpected turn.

PART II

RELATING TO CANCER

FOUR

Dancing With Cancer

QUESTIONS ASKED AND ANSWERED

About a week after I received my diagnosis, Pacific Urology called with the date and time for my urethral biopsy. "Be there at 11:30 a.m. a week from Tuesday," the woman announced brightly. "Also, we're scheduling you for a pre-surgery consult with Dr. Hopkins for this coming Friday."

The world of medicine proceeds at a far more leisurely pace than you would expect from watching medical shows on television. In this fictional world, doctors are always immediately available, tests are conducted speedily, diagnoses are made quickly, and the crises are fully resolved in the space of a one-hour network drama. By contrast, in my case, it was now early February, five months since my worrisome symptom and almost three months after my first meeting with Dr. Hopkins. Now there would be another ten days before the urethral biopsy and at least a week—and probably two—before its results would be known. This excruciatingly slow medical pace was directly at odds with the racing anxiety I was feeling. Yes, I knew that prostate cancer was typically slowgrowing, and that even with an aggressive version of it like mine, a few extra weeks, or maybe even a few months, were not all that critical. For the doctors, however, having enough time to formulate the appropriate treatment plan was essential. All the books and Internet sites I had consulted repeatedly stressed the need for thorough evaluation and reflection before starting treatment. Yet I repeatedly felt I was stuck on a slow-motion ride that kept stopping, starting, and then suddenly stopping again. The sluggish pace of the medical process necessitated being a "patient" patient.

To say I was dreading the urethral biopsy would have been an understatement, although I was at least looking forward to the consult with Dr. Hopkins. It would be my first real opportunity to ask the questions that had surfaced during my research. I had already completed the bone scan and had been taking the anti-androgen medication for a couple of months. Fortunately, I had noticed few side effects so far. However, the cancer diagnosis itself had really affected me psychologically. When awakening in the middle of the night to make the usual bathroom visits, it was now virtually impossible to fall right back to sleep, as I had been able to do so easily most of my life. In the 3:30 a.m. darkness, I rehearsed several highly imaginative but improbable scenarios, each with a really poor outcome. In the middle of the night, the high survival rate of prostate cancer and other optimistic statistics didn't seem to matter; dark fantasies ran rampant. As I would try to go back to sleep, I'd often think about which hymns I'd want to be played at my memorial service. Happily, daylight exposed the improbability of these scenarios, and the California morning sun would usually brighten my spirits.

On the day of the pre-surgery consult, Susan and I arrived early only to learn that Pacific Urology frequently double-booked its appointment calendar. We waited more than an hour before being ushered back to Dr. Hopkins's office. In his defense, he had always taken as much time as needed with me, so it was difficult to resent the time he spent with other patients. Given the significant nature of what we were about to discuss, I certainly didn't want to have the feeling he was watching the clock too closely.

In anticipation of our meeting, Susan and I had formulated a few "big questions" for the doctor. What specific data led to his diagnosis? How severe was my cancer's stage classification? What were the most critical next steps that needed to be taken? And, of course, the question I had framed during my information-gathering sessions on the Internet: How could I have had such consistently low PSA readings but still end up with aggressive cancer? Not that it mattered all that much now, but a number of friends who were comfortable with their own "normal" PSA levels had become understandably nervous when they heard my news. I wanted to have something valid and reassuring to say to them.

"Craig, you have a nasty cancer," Dr. Hopkins began. "It's probably locally advanced, which means it has penetrated the prostate capsule, but it has probably not yet spread to any other organs. We call that clinical stage T3."

Dr. Hopkins's estimate of clinical stage T3 (the "T" stands for tumor) offered greater precision than the word "nasty," but I now understood why he chose to use that particular adjective. I definitely harbored something more ominous than a run-of-the-mill cancer languidly growing inside my prostate gland. Since we met last, he had definitely revised his original assessment, abandoning the idea that my cancer was "localized," or fully contained in my prostate. The Gleason score of 8 meant it was aggressive, sometimes called "highgrade." The stage designation, T3, meant the cancer was already outside my prostate, poised—if it had not done so already—to invade nearby organs, especially lymph nodes and bones. While he did not say so, I suspected his assessment was based on what he saw in my urethra during the cysto—and that he wished to perform the urethral biopsy to confirm his suspicion. Accepting that I had prostate cancer was one thing, but the fact that my cancer was worthy of adjectives like "high grade," "aggressive," and "fastgrowing" took my breath away.

"The important thing right now is that you continue to take the anti-androgen meds so we can slow the cancer's growth. That will give us time to work out the other treatment steps," the doctor continued. "I'm concerned about the lesion on your urethra that I saw during the cystoscopy. That's why I want to do the urethral biopsy next week. It may be related to the prostate cancer, or it may be something completely different. In any event, we need to go in and look," he said.

"So, after the biopsy, what happens next?" Susan asked. "This whole process seems to be taking an awfully long time," she said, expressing the anxiety that we both felt about the slow pace at which events seemed to be unfolding.

"Well, we've already started Craig on the anti-androgen drugs almost a month ago. We need to give them time to shrink his prostate," he replied. "We'll be able to discuss some treatment options at our next meeting. By then, we'll have the results of the urethral biopsy and the data from the bone scan."

"But I thought I already had the bone scan," I interjected. "I was just about to ask you about the results."

"Well, embarrassingly enough, I checked the wrong box on the lab form, and you actually received a bone density test, instead. Now, as it turns out, it's a good thing you had that density test. You have osteopenia, which is a precursor to osteoporosis."

"Great," I exclaimed. "You mean there's still more wrong with me? What does this have to do with the prostate cancer?"

"It's independent of the cancer. Some people have the condition, some don't. What's important though is that to keep your bones strong you'll need to do resistance exercise like weights and stretching. And you'll need to take lots of calcium and Vitamin D."

Cancer was apparently not sufficient punishment, I thought darkly. Even my bones were screwed up. All those years I had spent jogging, going to the gym, and working out suddenly felt like a giant waste of time.

"We still need you to have a bone scan to make sure the cancer has not spread to your pelvis. I'm fairly sure it hasn't, but we need to verify that," Dr. Hopkins said, pulling my thoughts back to the conversation at hand.

By this time, most of my questions had been answered. I mentally toted up the score: Gleason 8 high-grade cancer, which was comparatively aggressive and fast growing. Clinically, the tumor was stage T3, which indicated it had escaped the prostate and was headed to nearby organs and/or lymph nodes. Oh, and I also had osteopenia of the bones, meaning I was prone to osteoporosis. But at least we had started treatment with the anti-androgen drugs, which should slow down the cancer's growth. One big question remained.

"So, how can I have a low PSA and aggressive cancer at the same time?" I asked.

"It doesn't happen very often, but the cells of an aggressive or high-grade cancer like yours are poorly differentiated, that is, they are not formed like disciplined, healthy prostate cells.

Instead, they have formed very haphazard—almost random— cell structures. When the cancer cells are so dissimilar to healthy prostate cells, the cancer cells simply do not express much, if any, of the prostate-specific antigen enzyme, so the PSA level remains low."

A few weeks later, I found a relevant paper at the National Cancer Institute website confirming his explanation. The paper stated, "In one large study prostate cancer was diagnosed in 15.2 percent of men with a PSA level at or below 4.0 ng/mL. Fifteen percent of these men, or approximately 2.3 percent overall, had high-grade [aggressive] cancers."

So, I was apparently the "lucky" one out of forty-four men diagnosed with prostate cancer who had this unfortunate combination of seemingly "normal PSA" and an aggressive cancer. Usually, I would have enjoyed an opportunity to stand out from my peers. But this particular distinction was one I could have done without.

"When we meet to discuss the urethral biopsy results in a couple of weeks, we can talk about the best course of treatment," Dr. Hopkins said, as he began intentionally to wrap things up.

Susan interjected, "At this point, what do you think those might be?"

"Probably radiation or surgery or both," he replied.

So there they were: the possible treatment methods for my case. By this time, I had pretty much accepted the reality of my cancer. Today I had learned the detailed information that had forced me to accept its severity. Now that the possible treatment options were on the table, I had definitely climbed aboard the Oncology Adventure Ride, and it was pulling away from the platform. Suddenly, I felt engulfed with that last-second panic that sometimes happens just before a roller coaster ride starts. I wanted nothing more than to unfasten the seatbelt and return to the safety of the platform before anything even scarier happened.

ANOTHER BIOPSY

The urethral biopsy, which was conducted at a local surgery center the following week, did not begin auspiciously. Clad only in a hospital gown and socks, I shivered both from nervousness and the relentless chill in the pre-op preparation room. The room's stark medical surroundings heightened my tension. The nurse tried to insert an IV in my left arm, but gave up after two unsuccessful tries. He called a second nurse, who after a single unsuccessful try on my right arm, finally asked for the most seasoned IV practitioner on duty to come over. "Shy veins," the experienced nurse stated authoritatively. She succeeded on her first attempt. I now had one IV and three bandages before the biopsy had even started.

Shortly thereafter, Dr. Hopkins arrived, dressed in his surgical scrubs. "Depending on how things go, you might wake up with a Foley urinary catheter in place," he counseled. Following his visit came a briefing by the anesthesiologist, who made me truly grateful that this procedure was being conducted under general anesthesia. Shortly after, I climbed into a wheelchair and was rolled into the operating room. After climbing on to the hard, narrow operating table, I saw Dr. Hopkins, the anesthesiologist, and a nurse hovering overhead. An oxygen mask was placed over my face. No one even asked me to count backward.

There was a loud rushing noise in the midst of the blackness. The noise gradually subsided and was replaced by mumbling voices. My visual field turned from black to gray and then I could see that I was in some sort of curtained enclosure. "Well, hi there." That voice I knew. It was Susan, welcoming my return to consciousness.

A different voice advised, "Take your time. We'll stay right here." The same nurse who had successfully started my IV was standing next to Susan.

Slowly emerging from gray disorientation, I became aware of my body. I felt no pain. Susan told me later that I was flying high on a morphine-based painkiller. A tube emerging from under the sheet confirmed that I had indeed been outfitted with a catheter.

I only have only a hazy memory of the ride home, but I remember Susan saying that I was in the operating room for about ninety minutes and that she had a lengthy discussion with Dr. Hopkins afterward. Apparently he had discovered a lot of unusual material in my urethra. Susan asked him whether or not it was cancerous. He had avoided answering directly, estimating that there was about a 50 percent chance that the pathologist would find that the material was malignant. In the days before we received the results of the biopsy, I focused on the 50 percent chance that it was benign.

A few weeks after my diagnosis, I had started keeping a journal. Journaling was a new experience for me, and it turned out to be therapeutic: Writing my thoughts as they occurred was a markedly different experience than writing the hundreds of memos, emails, reports, technical essays, brochure copy, and PowerPoint presentations that I had produced over the course of my career. There was something about writing that made helped me make sense of my jumbled thoughts, thereby reducing my general anxiety.

Two days after the urethral biopsy I wrote:

"I suppose I should start coming to grips with my feelings about where things stand now. Even though I'm resolved to take things one day at a time, and lean more heavily on my faith, on Susan, and on my friends, I still find myself strangely detached from the reality of what is happening. Many things continue normally as they always have: working, photography, reading the paper, watching TV with Susan in the evenings. But there are new, scarier things, too: being sucked into the maw of medical process. Devoting entire days to 'procedures.' A general sense of foreboding that seems especially real about 2:00 a.m. I keep trying to tell myself that I will come out of the other end of all this unscathed, and things will be pretty much the same as before. Yet, deep down, a bunch of things will be different. What are those things? How will I feel about these changes?"

A MATTER OF RELATIONSHIP

I now see that journal entry as my first honest attempt to come to terms with the new relationship that had entered unbidden into my life. Strangely, the one feeling I had supposed would dominate all others had not occurred. I felt no anger, no fury, no outrage toward my cancer. As my journal noted, I felt only detachment. Even though cancer had already altered much of my daily routine, the disease itself still felt unreal and far away. Deep down, I knew this detachment was probably transitory. I had been thrust into a new bond with an intimate partner that I could not ignore. But how does one establish a meaningful relationship with an uninvited intruder?

One thing seems clear: The nature and course of the disease—its personality, if you will—play an enormous role in defining the connection between its host and itself. Some cancers are so virulent and move so quickly that there may be no time to contemplate one's relationship with the disease. These highly aggressive—and inevitably incurable—carcinomas are analogous to an abusive marriage. The cancer takes on the cruelty of an overbearing spouse who so dominates the relationship that the weaker partner effectively disappears from view. In the end, it is not a relationship at all; it is a conquest. Al, a long-time leader at my church, was diagnosed with Stage IV lung cancer just two months before succumbing to it. The disease simply dominated every aspect of his life from his initial diagnosis to his death. It was pointless for him to think about how he would come to terms with his cancer. He barely had time to put his worldly affairs in order.

On the other hand, prostate cancer is relatively slow growing (although not always that slow growing, as in my case), with a high survival rate, so there's almost always sufficient time to think about how to relate to the disease that has invaded one's body. Each man has to choose how to imagine his cancer as a companion, and his vision will be shaped, in part, by his particular personality and circumstances. When I was diagnosed, I brought my passion to understand the rational "whys," constantly seeking out more information about my cancer, its course, its treatment, and its possible consequences. Other men may bring a peaceful acceptance, defeated resignation, or they may face the invader as an enemy with an aggressive stance, ready to do battle to the end. Many others may choose to ignore the cancer as best they can, deciding simply to "get through it," come out the other end of treatment and move on with life, never looking back. For them, it's as if the cancer never happened. But of course it did.

A man's relationship to his cancer will also depend on the nature of the disease itself. Someone diagnosed with a localized prostate cancer, one that's contained completely within the prostate capsule itself, will experience a different connection to his cancer than another man diagnosed with a Stage IV malignancy that has already metastasized to other organs or, more commonly, to distant bones of his body. With some forms of slow-growing, localized prostate cancer, the best option in fact may be to leave it untreated, since the side effects of surgery or radiation can be often worse than the harm the tumor itself can cause. However, not everyone can live peacefully with the knowledge that he has a tumor growing inside him, which leads many men to choose to remove the cancer without fully considering the consequences of surgery or radiation.

For younger and healthier men with localized prostate cancer, surgery is the most popular treatment option. However, surgery can have long-term effects on urinary function and sexual performance. Nerve-sparing surgery with laparoscopic and robotic technologies have somewhat reduced these concerns in the past several years. Nevertheless, fear of potential side effects causes many men to forego surgery, opting instead for other therapies such as brachytherapy (which implants radioactive seeds into the prostate) or electron beam radiotherapy (about which I will write more later). But none of these treatment options is free of potentially life-altering effects.

Treatment choices for a man with locally advanced cancer are fewer, and so his relationship with cancer is different. Surgery may be inappropriate, leaving only hormone therapy and/or one of the several forms of radiotherapy as the remaining treatment options. A man with metastasized Stage IV prostate cancer has an even more constrained set of treatment choices, none of them pleasant. It often begins with hormone therapy, and when that almost inevitably fails, there will be "second line" hormone treatments, possibly immunotherapy and eventually chemotherapy, frequently accompanied by external beam radiation to reduce pain in the bone "mets" that typically characterize metastasized prostate cancer. But, by definition, metastasized cancer cannot be put back into the box and leads only one direction, although perhaps years down the line.

Like a marriage, each individual union of a man with his disease has a different dynamic. If the man with Stage II cancer elects surgery, and the clinical "T" staging was correct, the relationship ends in simple divorce. The malignancy is removed right along with the prostate. Post-surgery, this man will always be a cancer survivor, but as one important study concluded, he has basically ended his day-to-day relationship with his disease.

My friend Denny, in his mid-50s, called me two days before my urethral biopsy. He described his encounter with prostate cancer and his surgery two years previously to remove it. The surgery for his T2, Gleason 6 carcinoma was successful, and he recovered fully within six months. "I just wanted to say that this cancer is survivable and not as bad as some people have made it out to be," he said encouragingly. Here was a man who had divorced his cancer, happy that his relationship with the disease lay firmly in his past. However, my aggressive Gleason 8 cancer had most likely escaped my prostate gland. This meant that I would have a different experience with my disease than Denny had with his. I just didn't know quite yet what that experience would be. Had my cancer already taken the upper hand in our relationship? Did Dr. Hopkins know more than he had already indicated to Susan and me? The urethral biopsy was a full-fledged surgical procedure involving general anesthesia. Surely, he wouldn't have performed that if he didn't already suspect the cancer had migrated there.

THE NEXT PIECE OF THE PUZZLE

The interval between the urethral biopsy and the scheduled "results meeting" with Dr. Hopkins felt like the longest two weeks of my life. Susan and I tempered the anxiety of the wait with a trip to Southern California and a delightful performance at the Los Angeles Philharmonic. For one evening, at least, my health was blessedly far from our thoughts. We were reminded that life continues without having to put cancer at the front and center of every waking moment.

From L.A., we drove up to the central California coast, north of Big Sur. Once again, we visited the beauty of the Point Lobos Reserve, where the sky, sea, woods, and rocks meet in unsurpassed drama. We had fallen in love with Point Lobos and, yes, with each other, on a bright July afternoon more than forty years before. This place has become one of those fixed points that help define relationships, and to which we return almost every year: the same paths, the same beaches, and the same relentless crash and retreat of water on rock. The gnarled shapes of the Monterey Cypress that cling to the steep cliffs appeared unaffected by forty intervening winters. Yes, there were probably some meaningful life lessons for us here about surviving life's storms, but happily, cancer was too far from our minds to grasp them at that particular moment.

The waiting room at Pacific Urology features a flat screen television that endlessly replays a DVD of the documentary *Planet Earth*. My previous visits involved substantial waiting before being called, so by this time, I had seen most of the documentary, albeit in discontinuous fragments spread across several months. After I once again watched the mountain goats climb the Himalayas, Susan and I were called into Dr. Hopkins's office.

"Well, the good news," he began, "is that you've responded nicely to the anti-androgen medication. Your PSA has dropped to 0.75. Also, the bone scan is clear.

"The less good news is that the biopsy shows that the prostate cancer has spread to your urethra."

Well, so much for the 50 percent chance of the lesion's being benign, I thought.

"Does prostate cancer invade the urethra very often?" I asked.

"No, it's really quite rare. Prostate cancer usually heads for the bladder; yours traveled in the opposite direction."

"So, what does this mean for the treatment options?" queried Susan.

"Well, surgery would be a bad option. And I'm a surgeon."

Wearily, I noted to myself that he put it more positively than saying, "Craig, you have inoperable cancer."

"If we operated, we couldn't get all the cancer," Dr. Hopkins continued. "We'd have to remove your sphincter, and you know what that means." I did. There was no need to utter the words, "permanent incontinence."

"There's really only one course I'd recommend: to stay on the anti-androgen hormone therapy together with a 9-week course of radiation. I'm going to refer you to Dr. Vincent Massullo, who is the head radiation oncologist over at John Muir Hospital."

He picked up the phone and called Dr. Massullo. Quickly lapsing into doctor-speak, he described my case. "Hi, Vince. Say, I've got a fellow here with multifocal Gleason 8 prostate cancer. It's a urethral lesion of necrotic tissue in the area of the sphincter, distal to the prostatic urethra." They engaged in some further logistic details, including him saying rather mysteriously, "I'll have Craig come over and pick up the gold seeds." Then he hung up.

It was oddly intriguing to hear my medical condition described in "doctor speak." But there it was: the official diagnosis in the official jargon. By the definition used by the National Cancer Institute, the fact the cancer had migrated to another organ—in this case, my urethra—technically raised my cancer tumor staging from T3 to T4. But, the cancer was still considered "locally advanced," since it was confined to my urological system; it had not metastasized to other regions of my body, at least as far as anyone could tell.

A Note on Cancer Staging

Staging is how the world of oncology estimates the extent of a cancer. For prostate cancer, "clinical staging" is the doctor's best estimate of how far it has spread, based on lab tests, cystoscopies, ultrasound probes, the biopsy, and the digital rectal exam—all in lieu of actually seeing the cancer first hand.

Cancer staging assesses the extent of tumor itself, whether or not lymph nodes are involved and whether or not the cancer has metatasized. The TNM system, consisting of descriptions of the extent of the tumor (T), amount, if any, of lymph node involvement (N), whether or not it has appeared in distant parts of the body (Distant metastasis [M]), and the histopathologic grade (G), which in the case of prostate cancer is the Gleason score. In turn, the American Joint Committee on Cancer (AJCC) staging system uses the TMN data to describe the over extent of cancer progression ranging from least severe (Stage I) to the most severe (Stage IV).

More information about staging of prostate cancer is available at The National Cancer Institute, which has a helpful Factsheet: *Staging Questions and Answers*, http://www.cancer.gov/cancertopics/factsheet/detection/staging, and a more technical description can be found at: http://www.cancer.gov/cancertopics/pdq/treatment/prostate/HealthProfessional/page4#Section_39

Dr. Hopkins continued, "I'm going to order an MRI to image the cancer that is outside your prostate. Also, you will need to stop by the Radiation Oncology Center over at John Muir and pick up four gold marker seeds that I am going to implant in your prostate. Those will serve as reference points for the radiation equipment."

As Dr. Hopkins stood up, signaling the end of the meeting, Susan boldly voiced the question that was clearly the elephant in the room, the one I could not bring myself to ask, "So what's Craig's prognosis?"

"We don't give prognoses," he replied blandly, "but we're going to work toward a cure." Dr. Hopkins had meant to convey encouragement, but my mood was dark. At the moment, I was not feeling particularly comforted by his reply.

COMING TO GRIPS

At last I had a lucid, if rather ominous, picture of my cancer's personality: Gleason 8, T4 locally advanced prostate cancer that had spread in an unusual direction to invade my urethra near my sphincter. I now had all the technical information I needed to figure out how I was going to engage in the relationship with my disease. But having the technical information was not enough. I needed to decide how to respond emotionally and psychologically to my new reality.

I really had three choices when it came to defining my relationship to my cancer. I could a) ignore (or, at least, try to ignore) the cancer; b) let cancer embrace me; or c) choose to embrace cancer.

So, how about the first option: just ignoring it? Unless it migrates to some nearby bone, prostate cancer is symptom free, even an aggressive cancer like mine. Other than the blood in my urine, my cancer had offered no overt sign of its presence, nor had it caused any pain. Unlike breast cancer, where an unexpected lump may be felt physically by self-examination, prostate cancer is impossible to self-diagnose. Elevated PSA levels can offer clues to prostate cancer's possible existence, but not always, as had happened in my case. Prostate cancer can be confirmed only by a needle biopsy—an undertaking that most men are happy to (and probably should) avoid until absolutely necessary.

Contrary to the sense of urgency that surrounds many other cancers, given the proper circumstances, ignoring—well, almost ignoring—prostate cancer can be a viable option. The majority of prostate cancers are slow growing, "indolent" in medical jargon. In 2006, the *Journal of the National Cancer Institute* published a study written by a team of urologists at Johns Hopkins Hospital that stated, "The risk of non-curable prostate cancer was the same for men receiving immediate surgical treatment and those who waited (on average) two years before surgery."

Translated into plain language, this means that many men with a low-grade, slow-growing prostate cancer can delay treatment without negatively affecting the ability to cure it later on. In fact, men who are diagnosed with prostate cancer in their 70s and beyond are statistically more likely to die of something other than their cancer. Since "ignoring it" is not on the list of approved terminology used by the medical community, postponing surgery, radiation, or other means of treating the cancer, is called "watchful waiting," "expectant management," or more recently, "active surveillance." According to one medical report, the clinical criteria for being able to watch the cancer without intervening—at least for a few years, anyway—are a Gleason score of less than or equal to 6, less than three biopsy cores containing cancer, and less than 50 percent cancer involvement of any core, together with regular PSA tests and annual biopsies. One study noted that, "Expectant management is still appropriate for elderly patients and patients who have significant co-morbidities such that life expectancy is less than ten years."

I wasn't even close to falling into the "expectant management" category. I had a high-grade, fast-growing tumor, and I was a relatively young 62 years old (at least to the medical world, which considers an age of less than 70 to be "young"). I also did not have any life-threatening co-morbidities such as heart disease or diabetes. In a way, it was a relief that active surveillance was off the table. I would not have been comfortable knowing a cancerous tumor was growing inside me, even if the medical community had given me a recommendation to leave it alone. I understood why many men resist active surveillance: Emotion often trumps the rational choice.

My second option was to allow cancer to dominate my life. This would have been easy to do. After all, that was pretty much what had happened so far. When I lapsed into this dark mode, my mind focused on how unfair the whole situation was. Why didn't my primary care doctor catch this when I had my annual physical just eight months previously? Surely there must have been some clue. Dr. Hopkins's comment that he could have caught it earlier certainly didn't reassure me about the medical care I'd been receiving up to this point—at least as far as my prostate was concerned. Why hadn't someone suggested continuing visits to Dr. Hopkins after my bout with prostatitis and a diagnosis of PIN seven years ago? In the end, though, I really had no one to blame but myself. Why hadn't I been more aggressive as an informed consumer and demanded regular follow-up visits? Why did I have to end up with the Gleason 8 T4 tumor? Why me? My brooding swirled downward into the depths of self-pity. But even in this blackest of emotional states, a tiny bit of my rational self remained. I realized that the moment I succumbed to "why me?" was the moment I would become a cancer victim, a helpless bystander overwhelmed by a relentless enemy.

The means by which cancer triumphs over its prey lies in more than just its physical qualities. Psychologically and emotionally, cancer inevitably becomes the center of the victim's universe, eclipsing everyone and everything else in his or her life. Virulent, often painful cancers that invade and eventually disable vital organs such as the brain, lungs, liver, and pancreas are especially skilled at this. The sufferer's world shrinks to "cancer and me," or perhaps more accurately, to "cancer and what used to be me." Virtually every waking moment is devoted to dealing with the carcinoma and its effects: waiting for appointments; undergoing invasive, often painful tests; receiving chemotherapy over a period of weeks and even months; dealing with insurance companies and hospital billing departments; and finally, putting one's affairs in order. There is barely time to carry out the regular tasks of daily life. Sleep, if it can be attained, is fitfully shallow.

Cancer is a selfish and jealous companion. It is not content just taking over the body. It works to supplant every other activity its victim once enjoyed. It prefers not to allow loving relationships to continue, although many do. But too often, even the deepest, strongest relationships become shells of their former selves. Oh, yes, other people still love the cancer victim, and they want to do everything they can to help. But cancer deadens the victim's feelings. It feeds not only on the body, but also on the psyche, and finally, on the victim's very identity. Cancer triumphs when the individual's name becomes synonymous with "cancer victim." Both print and electronic media outlets provide ample proof of this phenomenon in their headlines:

"Cancer victim's widow sues village ..."

"A cancer victim refuses chemotherapy."

"Cancer victim found dead."

"Students perform play in honor of cancer victim."

It would be easy to become a cancer victim, to let the disease throw its suffocating cape over me, to overwhelm my relationship with Susan, with my children and grandchildren, with my extended family, and with my friends. But even during my moments of deepest self-pity, I still hung on to a small resolve to be something other than cancer's victim. I had to summon a determination to choose the third course: not to ignore the cancer, not to be its victim, but to embrace it, and, yes, to own it, lest it own me.

DANCING WITH CANCER

By any measure, I am an ordinary man. Cancer unexpectedly entered my ordinary life. Even with my fairly unusual case, prostate cancer itself is, well, routine. In 2009, I joined upwards of two hundred thousand other American men diagnosed with prostate cancer. After completing treatment, I have now become a cancer survivor, although some argue that one is not a "survivor" until five years of cancer-free living have passed. Regardless of its definition, a survivor is a wonderful thing to be. The first Sunday of each June is National Cancer Survivors Day®. One can purchase tee shirts online that proclaim "Cancer Survivor!" The American Cancer Society sponsors and maintains the Cancer Survivors Network on the Internet with individual discussion forums for twenty-four different types of cancer. Lance Armstrong's foundation, LIVESTRONG has made the yellow wristbands celebrating cancer survivorship ubiquitous.

I am delighted to be a cancer survivor. But I am still left with the nagging feeling that the word "survivor" is insufficient to encompass all the dimensions of my ongoing relationship with cancer. Survivor implies a fixed goal of eventual achievement:

I was treated for cancer and came out the other side as a survivor. An authentic relationship, on the other hand, is a dynamic, ongoing process, not just the achievement of a single static goal, however worthy.

So, how does one go about "owning" cancer? Many metaphors might work. The most popular one is military: We "battle cancer." We become cancer "warriors." But both words imply the possibility that cancer could win the war. That's always a possibility, maybe even an inevitability, but "battle" certainly does not connote "ownership." Other men may turn to sports analogies. However, cancer is not a team sport, so the usual football and baseball metaphors fail. A marathon might work. Prostate cancer is definitely a long race, and physical collapse near the finish line is always a possibility. Others may prefer the analogy of a wrestling match. This image certainly captures the idea of foes opposing each other, but I'm not sure being locked in a tight, permanent embrace with cancer conveys the sense of the honest relationship between equals that I was seeking.

The metaphor that best encompasses my personal relationship with cancer is ballroom dancing. Dancing is both a sport and an art. On the dance floor, it takes two parties to comprise the whole. I am cancer's partner, its equal. It requires adroitness and mastering a wide variety of different moves. There are times when the partners are holding each other in a tight embrace. There are other times when they are farther apart, dancing in synchronicity, or sometimes dancing in contrast, against one another.

The most important quality of this metaphor, though, is that the partners are engaged in a constantly changing dynamic relationship. Some days it seems as if the cancer is breathing right over my shoulder, ready to grab me at the first sign of weakness. Other days, the cancer will be farther away, and I'm dancing solo, with my partner somewhere outside my line of sight. But I must always remember that it has never left the ballroom floor.

Cancer and I danced arm in arm during the months of treatment. We will continue to dance close to each other for the remainder of my life, as I continue with hormone treatments, nervously wait for the results of the frequent PSA tests that will tell me if the cancer has returned. But at other times, I will be dancing free, virtually alone. The shadow of the cancer always remains, but there will be moments when the spotlight is only on me. At those times, I remain the man I always was.

My former boss and mentor, Ron Borrelli, was the best dancer I have ever known. Not on the actual ballroom floor, although I watched him dance the waltz with fatherly affection at each of his four daughters' weddings. More importantly, Ron danced a superlative waltz with cancer. The first occasion was with a carcinoma in his left arm in the early 1990s. The treatment for that cancer involved microsurgery and radioactive needles inserted painfully into his muscle. The cancer never slowed him down, though. Ron recovered sufficient use of his arm and was able to resume his beloved tennis game. Just a few years later, he was diagnosed with prostate cancer. This was the first time I'd heard of a robotic prostatectomy, but Ron was an early adopter of new technology, always willing to try something new. The surgery was successful, and he recovered fully. In the summer of 2007, just after completing a tennis game, Ron experienced a significant memory lapse and became confused about where he was. His diagnosis was swift and devastating: glioblastoma, a highly aggressive brain tumor. Still, he danced willingly, undertaking a rigorous course of radiotherapy. When I last visited Ron, he described his symptoms at length, completely aware of the various brain and speech functions he had already lost—and the ones he was about to lose in a matter of weeks. The last thing we talked about was the renovation he was doing to his patio and the beautiful new waterfall that would be there. Susan and I left his house that day with Ron eagerly planning for the future. He died a couple of months later. Ron was no Pollyanna awash in overoptimistic or unrealistic scenarios. From his first diagnosis in 1992 to his death in 2007, Ron danced with cancer: sometimes very close, sometimes farther away. With the brain cancer, he knew his chances of a full recovery were extremely small, but he never became a victim. Instead, he forcefully owned his cancer by first accepting its reality and then always looking ahead to the future.

Our unique ability as human beings—to anticipate and to plan—is what it means to dance with cancer. We need to acknowledge that the disease changes our lives, but then we need to look ahead with undimmed anticipation to what comes next. For me, that is the essence of my dance with cancer—and to my decision to own it, instead of allowing it own me.

FIVE

Speaking of Cancer

TO SPEAK OR HOLD MY TONGUE?

Even though I might learn to dance with my cancer, there was still the question of the audience in the ballroom: all the people in my life. This group ranged from my family and close friends to professional contacts and casual acquaintances.

In addition to defining his relationship to his cancer itself, each man must decide if—and how—he will discuss his disease with the people in his life. If he decides to talk with others about his cancer, he'll probably want to have as much control as possible over how that happens. Inevitably, he will still be coming to terms with the fact that he has cancer when he must undertake the difficult task of deciding what to share and with whom. This is not easy.

I began to talk about my cancer the moment I blurted out, "I have prostate cancer" to Susan. Over the next few days, however, I began to wonder whether talking so openly to others was really a wise decision. Perhaps keeping the details of my situation more discreet would simplify things. After all, I had a rough road ahead. Why should I waste my limited energy figuring out what to tell others? The default position for many men is to say little, if anything, to anyone. As I considered how and when to communicate my bad news, I found there are numerous ways to justify staying silent about cancer—some cultural, some personal.

CULTURAL SILENCE

Our culture has slowly become one of over-sharing. We now rarely hesitate to talk about many issues once considered private: goals, worries, psychoses, drugs, bad habits, and of course, sex. Every conceivable topic has become fair game for discussion, analysis, and dissection, and we share these thoughts and feelings through multiple media sources. Little is thought to be private anymore. But how comfortable have people been with talking about disease, especially cancer? At first glance, it seems the discussion is everywhere. The media lose little time to inform us when a celebrity has breast, lung, or pancreatic cancer. Tobacco suit money funds gruesome TV spots that remind us of the dangers of smoking, clearly implying cancer will not be far behind. But at a personal level, few people would tell a random passerby on the street about their cancer.

Nor can newly-diagnosed men look to the previous generation for guidance on how to speak openly about prostate cancer. Compared to the "Greatest Generation" born in the 1920s and 1930s, even the most reticent men today appear talkative and open. The Depression-bred attitude of "keeping one's chin up" applied to more than financial issues. This was the era when many men dressed for work and left the house each morning, even though their unemployment gave them nowhere to go. Appearances were important. This was the same cohort of men that fought the "necessary war" explored by Tom Brokaw in his book, *The Greatest Generation Speaks*. In an interview with Larry King, Brokaw notes, "They didn't want to talk about their experiences because they knew other people were going through something that was more difficult."

In the years before World War II, illness, like so many other topics, was strictly a personal matter—and no disease was more private than cancer. My mother remembered that as a young girl, she inadvertently walked in on a whispered conversation between her mother and grandmother about a neighbor woman who had been diagnosed with breast cancer. At least this is what she assumed, since both women stopped speaking as soon as she entered the room. Cancer was not a topic to be discussed in polite society, and certainly not in front of children.

Like many other aging members of that generation, LeRoy, a distant relative of mine, was diagnosed with prostate cancer in his mid-80s. He remained firmly committed to not discussing his disease with anyone. In 2009, LeRoy's widow recalled that he was barely able to utter the words "prostate cancer" to her, and he refused to share with his friends and family—including his son—the details of his condition. He underwent 43 sessions of radiation, driving to and from the hospital by himself every day. For LeRoy, having cancer was a private matter.

PSYCHOLOGICAL SILENCE

We men, many of us already culturally predisposed not to discuss disease of any kind, much less cancer, have other personal justifications to remain silent. Much of our reluctance may have to do with our attitude toward our bodies. Discussing diseases that affect our sexual organs is not for the socially squeamish. Prostate cancer and its treatments often compromise a man's sexual ability, and often his urinary and bowel functions as well. And if a man's prostate cancer is treated with "hormone therapy"—the less euphemistic term is "chemical castration"—the feelings of shame and inadequacy may be more intense.

Yvonne Hanson, an experienced marriage and family therapist, believes that, "women are more open than men to discussing their sexual organs. Women are more comfortable with their bodies because of menstruation, which forces them into the reality of knowing their bodies from the time they're young girls. Boys and men simply haven't had to face these issues."

As proof of her thesis, Hanson observed, "In my experience, when a woman faces a hysterectomy she's much less hesitant to proceed with it than is a male thinking about a vasectomy, never mind something serious like prostate cancer. When I ask men questions about sexual issues during counseling sessions, I often get only 'uhhhh' as a response.

"Discussing erectile dysfunction (ED) is especially difficult for most men, although the recent rash of TV advertising about ED may be changing this," she continued. "As for older men I can't even ask questions about sexual issues. They simply won't answer.

"I believe a root cause of the difference in willingness to talk openly is that women are used to networking with other women from an early age. They are willing to learn how to help themselves, and are much more likely than men to seek community. Men are more naturally 'solo creatures,' and don't have as many opportunities—and many lack the skills—to network well.

"Happily, for younger men, this go-it-alone culture of isolating oneself is diminishing somewhat as tasks such as shared parenting and stay-at-home fathering become more prevalent."

When it comes to cancer, however, even younger men become reluctant to share their experiences. Hanson pointed out that the initial reaction to a cancer diagnosis is invariably fear, expressed as the natural first question, "Am I going to die?" Next follows, "What have I lost?" For men diagnosed with prostate cancer, the answer to the latter question almost always includes their sexual function, thereby creating feelings of shame. "And people invariably hide when they are feeling shame," Hanson asserted.

"Being treated for prostate cancer and its implications for loss of libido and sexual performance, as well as the possibility of incontinence are understandable sources of shame. The only way to overcome shame is to talk about its causes. Not talking can easily become a self-perpetuating circle of silence," she concluded.

Nor does the American medical system make it easier for men to speak up about their condition. One editorial in the *Journal of Urology,* commenting on the reluctance of men to even visit a health care provider in the first place, noted subtle barriers for men,

> *Embarrassment begins with registration with a female receptionist for a "male" complaint. ... Physicians' offices also tend to be "feminized" as exemplified by furniture, decorating and reading material.*

Choosing if and when to talk about a cancer diagnosis is a complex personal decision. So is choosing to remain silent. Often generational and cultural factors keep men from speaking out. Psychologically, men may also have a subliminal fear that talking about cancer makes it more real and therefore more dangerous. But staying silent also comes with a price.

My friend, Chuck, just a few years older than I, understands the long-term effects of remaining silent. He was diagnosed with colorectal cancer more than fifteen years ago while still in his early 50s. His case was fairly severe, and he had to endure surgery followed by courses of chemotherapy and radiation. Nevertheless, throughout more than a year of treatment, Chuck revealed little to others about his condition. His wife was aware of his disease, but he refused to talk to her about the details of his physical condition or his feelings about having cancer. He went to the hospital alone and underwent his outpatient treatments alone. No one came to visit him at the hospital, because no one knew he was there. Chuck's friends and co-workers were only vaguely aware that he was sick. A few acquaintances speculated that he might have cancer, but Chuck provided no verification. Eventually he recovered, but he never spoke about his ordeal, other than to say, "I was ill, but I'm better now."

When I asked Chuck why he didn't want to discuss his cancer, he said he felt he could handle it alone. Above all, he did not want his wife to worry any more than she had to. This is a common reason for not talking about cancer: a patient's desire to avoid causing further distress to loved ones. Many men believe, usually incorrectly, that remaining silent will reduce the anxiety of those around them.

Chuck's attitude has changed in the fifteen years since his diagnosis and treatment. When he learned of my diagnosis, the first thing he said was, "Don't do what I did, man. Don't keep it to yourself. It just eats away at you." He now believes that keeping silent was detrimental to his loved ones, especially his wife. "Keeping her in the dark did nothing to protect her from bad news. On the contrary, it only increased her anxiety and left her feeling cut off," Chuck explained.

In the end, whether to speak or to remain silent is a deeply personal decision. There is no clear right or wrong. For me, keeping silent was not the answer. For one thing, it would have required me to develop elaborate strategies as Chuck had done in order to hide my cancer's existence from others.

But once cancer patients decide to speak with other people, they have to figure out how to do it. As I learned, communicating with others about cancer can be fraught with complex emotions. While my decision to speak openly with others may have felt right to me, the next step in the process was not clear. Whom to tell? When to tell them? What details should I include? I hadn't thought this all through the first few times I shared my news.

On the morning I was diagnosed and had blurted out to Susan, "I have prostate cancer," we were on our way to a previously scheduled lunch with close friends, who already knew I had an appointment with Dr. Hopkins. Shortly after we sat down, they asked directly, "So, Craig how was your visit to the doctor?" My reply was immediate and direct, albeit less dramatic than my earlier announcement to Susan. For better or worse, and with no strategic plan in mind, I began down the path of sharing my story openly, trusting that the people I cared about would join me on my journey into the unknown.

ENTERING THE WORLD OF RADIATION ONCOLOGY

Before being able to reflect more about how and to whom to tell my story, the next stage in the Oncology Adventure Ride started up. I began to learn about the treatment method—electron beam radiotherapy (EBRT)—that Dr. Hopkins said would be the best course to treat my cancer. The physical reality of the Radiation Oncology Center of the John Muir Cancer Institute was in stark opposition to its grandiose name. "Rad onc," as it was universally known, was tucked away on the basement floor of a modest annex of the main hospital. Its entrance opened into a very cramped waiting area of just six chairs. A table against one wall was stocked with fresh fruit, drinks, and graham crackers. A second table held an enormous stack of magazines of indeterminate dates. Shortly after we arrived, Susan and I were escorted to a small exam room. After just a few minutes, a cheerful balding man of medium height entered the room, shook our hands, and introduced himself as Dr. Vincent Massullo. His warm smile and kind manner immediately calmed both of us. After brief introductory pleasantries, the doctor launched immediately into an explanation about the benefits of radiotherapy.

"The cure rate for prostate cancer is the same for surgery and radiation. Sixty percent of the men who have surgery turn out to have more disease than originally thought, which means they often have to do radiation and hormone therapy anyway," he said. It sounded as if he had given this speech to many men who were deeply disappointed to be sent over to radiation oncology because, like me, they were not candidates for surgery, or their surgery had disclosed a more widespread cancer than previously assumed, thereby requiring "salvage" radiation.

"The combination of hormone therapy and radiation is better than radiation alone and adds about 15 percent to the cure rate," he continued.

Dr. Massullo turned, looked directly at me, and said, "Craig, you are a rare case; very few men present with such a low PSA and such extensive cancer. We're going to go for broke. The course I'm recommending is the same one I did for my dad three years ago," quickly adding that his father was still very much alive.

"We'll start your radiation course on a machine using intensity-modulated radiotherapy (IMRT). It will have a relatively broad field that will include your prostate, urethra, and the surrounding tissue in order to attack possible lymph node involvement. Then, about two-thirds of the way through the course, you'll go on a different machine that uses what we call image-guided radiotherapy (IGRT). On this one, the radiation will be aimed only at your prostate gland. This is the machine that uses the gold seeds Dr. Hopkins told you about."

After entering a few keystrokes on his computer, he swiveled the monitor so it was facing us. It displayed the home page of a website maintained by the Memorial Sloan-Kettering Cancer Center in New York. "This site consists of an extensive database, together with a form where you can enter your 'numbers,' including PSA, Gleason score, number of cancerous cores detected in the biopsy, along with a few other inputs." Dr. Massullo explained. "It uses a mathematical tool called a nomogram that compares your numbers against the database and predicts the statistical probability of outcomes of different types of prostate cancer treatments for a person with your numbers."

After entering my data, he continued, "With the radiation therapy I'm recommending, you have a 93 percent probability that the cancer will not progress further within the five years following treatment."

There's a big difference between statistics based on a sizable group, and what can actually happen in each individual case. Nevertheless, a statistical 93 percent probability of being cancer-free after five years was encouraging. Next, Dr. Massullo changed the treatment option to surgery instead of radiation. This single alteration reduced the statistical likelihood of being cancer-free in five years to 76 percent—a much less desirable outcome than that predicted for radiation. His demonstration complete, Dr. Massullo turned to me and said, "Radiation definitely looks to be the best course for you, Craig."

This statistical difference of the probable outcomes between radiation and surgery was unsurprising. Since my cancer was "locally advanced," the odds of surgery removing every cancer cell floating around outside my prostate were much smaller than if the cancer had remained safely inside the gland itself. As someone who had worked in marketing for more than thirty years, I recognized the doctor's sales technique immediately: a convincing demonstration accompanied by the presumptive close that, of course, I would opt for a treatment regimen of radiotherapy. Although I suspected Dr. Massullo had employed this technique frequently, Susan and I were nevertheless reassured. The doctor then brought us back to the real world, noting, "There's also a 15 percent chance that there is already lymph node involvement. While that's not high, it's still significant." I felt my optimism receding again, so I changed the subject.

"Several people have suggested that I should go to Loma Linda for proton beam therapy. What's the story on that?" I asked. (Loma Linda is a medical center located in Southern California about 400 miles from my home in the San Francisco Bay Area.)

"Statistically," Dr. Massullo replied, "there's really no significant difference between proton beam and the intensity-modulated radiotherapy I'm recommending for you. Nor have there been any studies that have directly compared proton beam therapy with the newer radiotherapy techniques we use here at John Muir. Proton beam therapy has proven quite effective for children who have cancer, and for people with oddly shaped tumors. I have sent several people to Loma Linda for proton beam treatment. For your case, though, I think we can do an equally good job with our radiation techniques right here."

Frankly, I didn't really need that much convincing. Proton beam radiation might produce a slightly better outcome with fewer side effects, but for me, there would be a steep price of having to live for at least eight weeks in a motel room almost 400 miles away from my family and support system. That was something I was just not mentally, psychologically, or financially prepared for.

I moved on to a different question. "What's the process for getting the radiation treatment started?" Hearing words like "aggressive," "high-grade," and "advanced" had made me anxious to start treating this cancer as soon as possible.

"We start with simulation," he replied.

"Simulation of what?" I asked.

"We develop an individual treatment plan for each patient that places the right amounts of radiation at precisely the right locations in your body. We need to have as much data as possible about your anatomy. We use a CT scan system to collect specific information about your body. We then take the simulation data and any other scans you have, such as the MRI that Dr. Hopkins has already ordered for you. With all the imaging data in hand, we develop the actual dosing program that's used by our computer-controlled radiotherapy equipment," he explained. "It takes about two weeks from the simulation to the beginning of the actual radiation therapy."

I had spent my engineering and marketing career among computer-controlled equipment used for testing semiconductors and electronic circuit boards, so I understood the process to which he was referring. However, my in-depth knowledge of computer-controlled machines was also a disadvantage, since I was well aware of the numerous things that can go wrong during the programming process. Incorrectly programmed test equipment can destroy the chips or circuit boards these systems are supposedly testing. Since this was my body we were talking about, I definitely wanted a clear answer to my next question.

"Once you've developed the treatment program how do you check to make sure it's correctly programmed?"

"We run the program on the equipment without you there and measure the intensity and positioning of the dosing against the X-rays and scans we made during the simulation," he responded.

During our meeting that had lasted more than an hour, I had grown to really like Dr. Massullo with his mix of friendliness, expertise, frankness, and reassurance. He had been willing to take as much time as we needed with him, not only to answer our questions, but also to provide a realistic perspective about what lay ahead—both the positive and the negative. I left that day pretty much convinced that radiation was the right course to follow. Now, I just wanted to get on with it as soon as possible.

IN SICKNESS AND IN HEALTH

Riding a roller coaster with your friends is more fun than riding alone. There's something about shared anxiety that creates a tighter bond. Everything that I had discovered about the Oncology Adventure Ride confirmed that this was definitely not something I wanted to experience by myself. Underlying everything, of course, was the relationship—the dance I was choreographing—between my cancer and myself. But my relationships with other people were also critically important. Yes, I was already telling people that I had cancer, but now it was time to figure out how my cancer would affect my relationships. Which bonds might be put at risk if I didn't pay attention and allowed cancer to dominate my life?

All the information that I had read so far covered the medical and technical aspects of prostate cancer diagnosis and treatment. But I had found virtually nothing that spoke to cancer's impact on the important relationships in the male patient's life, especially the one with his wife or significant other. Articles written by women who had breast cancer were the only ones I had found so far that discussed how cancer affects relationships. One woman recently wrote a book about her husband's experience with prostate cancer. I also found a woman's blog about prostate cancer that included a few entries about relationships. Both were interesting, but both reflected the wife's point of view. The men who had been diagnosed with cancer seemed to be silent. Other blogs written by men with prostate cancer seemed to focus almost exclusively on its clinical aspects. These are admittedly important, but more medical facts were not what I was looking for right now. Apparently, I was going to have to figure out how to handle my personal connections pretty much on my own.

I started with my most significant and critical relationship, the one with my wife Susan. The year I was diagnosed with prostate cancer was the same year we had celebrated our fortieth wedding anniversary. Our relationship had been tested on that January morning in the Pacific Urology parking lot when I blurted out, "I have prostate cancer," with no attempt to deliver the news to Susan either gently or empathetically. During a conversation with therapist Yvonne Hanson, she suggested that the shock of my diagnosis had expressed itself as a subconscious need to shock the person closest to me.

Diagnosed with multiple sclerosis (MS) almost thirty years earlier, Susan had experience living with chronic illness. By comparison, I was a rank amateur. I had persuaded myself years before that I was sympathetic to the reality of her MS: that I fully appreciated the numbness in her limbs, the difficulty she had walking, and the fatigue—especially the fatigue. Now, I was quickly learning how little I had really understood. Just a couple of months into dealing with the impact of a diagnosis of cancer, I realized that what I had provided Susan all these years was assuredly not empathy; it was barely sympathy. A more accurate description of my attitude would be forbearance. Yes, I asked her from time to time how the MS made her feel, both physically and emotionally. Yes, I had made what I thought were some rather significant accommodations, such as consciously walking at her slower pace when we were on foot together. Up to now, MS had been the elephant in the room of our relationship as husband and wife: a looming presence I generally preferred to ignore as a topic of discussion. Moreover, I had acknowledged neither to her nor to myself just how much MS had actually impacted our relationship.

Granted, MS is a different disease with a different course than cancer, but they are similarly life altering. Now both of us had diseases that might remain in remission, or might advance unexpectedly to the next, more severe stage. Susan wrote of this uncertainty—with which she had lived for so long—in a heart-felt note that she gave me on Valentine's Day, a few weeks after my diagnosis.

> *"In sickness and in health." We sure never imagined this. Or rather, in our dumb, fat and happy days, we were able to think of ourselves as invincible ... or invulnerable ... or in control ... But here "it" is. Now we come face-to-face with our weakness and how little control we actually do have.*
>
> *Yet, there is one thing we can control: our love for one another. [Our] human love will give us strength for the journey ahead. As well, we will learn more to let the love of Jesus wash over us in ways that will surprise us.*

Her note left little doubt about how she viewed our relationship: Life is uncertain and we control far less than we imagine; yet life is exciting and all the richer for being able to experience each day together. Outwardly—my body, Susan's MS, our daily lives—appeared the much the same as before my diagnosis. But many of my long-held assumptions had to change. For as long as Susan had MS, both of us believed that she would be the care receiver and I—the presumptive healthy spouse—would be the caregiver. After all, I was the one who could go to work every day to provide for us. I was the one who could get the insurance policies. Now my cancer had turned comfortable assumptions like these on their heads. Much of our income came from my one-man marketing consulting business. I did not have sick or vacation pay. Every hour I did not—or could not—work was an hour of lost income. Even if I could stay well enough to work during treatment, there would still be big blocks of time during which I would be consumed with my medical care.

Beyond financial issues lurked another unknown: What about our physical relationship? Given the side effects of my treatment, what had previously been straightforward, age-related erectile dysfunction was now going to be something more—or more accurately, something far less. And what about our emotional relationship? How would our shared spiritual beliefs be impacted? Our marriage was about to be tested in ways that we had never imagined.

"For better or for worse, for richer, for poorer, in sickness and in health, to love and to cherish, from this day forward until death do us part." One evening, Susan provided me the reassurance that those vows we had made so many years ago would indeed hold true now. It had been a tiring day, and I sat at my desk reflecting darkly on our uncertain future. Susan came up behind me, leaned her head softly against mine and said simply, "I'll be here with you." Whatever came to pass, these words promised both of us that our journey was inextricably bound together. At that moment, "I'll be here with you" had an even deeper resonance than "I love you." For what Susan whispered in my ear was not merely an expression of love. It was love acted out.

GETTING THE WORD OUT

It was one thing for Susan and me to navigate the challenges of my cancer and her MS in our marriage, but there was still everyone else in my life to consider. Having decided that I would not keep my cancer a secret, I was surprised how challenging it was to decide how to share my diagnosis with others. I could have just posted "I have prostate cancer" on my Facebook page, but even in this era of uninhibited social networking, this strategy seemed foolish. After all, I was under no obligation to tell absolutely everyone I knew. While I was still emotionally raw about my diagnosis, I knew it would be in my best interest to communicate intentionally with those friends and acquaintances who were most likely to be supportive. It would be stressful—even demoralizing—to tell someone only to receive a response of polite indifference, or worse, no response at all.

My marketing experience led me to think about my "target audiences" and then to tailor my message appropriately to each group. Sorting family and friends by "audience" may seem coldly analytical, but it was a helpful way to craft an appropriate message for each group.

Shared beliefs and experiences form the basis of the stories we tell to each other. The words I used with my closest family and longstanding friends tended to be deeply personal, clearly exposing my feelings of vulnerability. I used a spiritual

My "target audiences" for discussing cancer

- Family
  - My adult children and their respective spouses
  - My parents, my brother, and my sister
  - Susan's siblings (and their spouses and families)
  - Other in-laws, e.g., my daughter-in-law's parents
- Friends
  - Friends who are themselves cancer survivors
  - Long-time friends with the same spiritual beliefs as I
  - Long-time friends absent an established spiritual context
- Casual acquaintances, including neighbors
- Clients and professional associates

framework and an appeal for prayers in telling the friends that I had known for years at my church. The message I conveyed to my clients and professional colleagues was as straightforward and as emotionally neutral as possible. Speaking with other cancer survivors was the easiest: They already "got it," having gone through the experience. In fact, what they had to say to me was usually more profound and valuable than anything I could say to them. I tried to do more listening than telling; we could almost communicate in shorthand.

The "how" part of the communication had two components. Wherever possible, I wanted to tell those closest to me one-on-one, preferably in person. But like many others of my age and background, my family, friends, colleagues, and casual acquaintances were spread across 12 time zones. Email became the indispensable medium. Susan was the first to send an email four days after my initial diagnosis, notifying her four siblings about me, using the subject line "not good news." Because of its ability to transcend time zones and geography, email quickly became the dominant medium Susan and I used to communicate with the entire range of target audiences. Between the time I was diagnosed and the end of the radiation course—a little over five months—we had sent and received more than 500 individual email messages.

As for the "what," I wanted the message to be as concise and straightforward as possible. My first email said simply, "I've been diagnosed with prostate cancer, and there isn't enough information yet to know what treatment I'll be undergoing or what the long-term prognosis is." The responses from our correspondents created what seemed to be an inexhaustible demand for more detailed information. So, rather than ignoring their pleas or just being cryptic, I decided to educate my friends and family about prostate cancer and its treatment. After all, I had known precisely nothing about prostate cancer when Dr. Hopkins first announced his diagnosis to me. Since most of my male friends were about my age, describing the specifics of what was happening could act also be helpful if they, too, someday faced a similar situation. If detailed descriptions of my experience encouraged the older men among them to be more diligent about having DREs and PSA tests, so much the better.

Two weeks following my diagnosis, I emailed a fairly thorough status report with the subject line "Where things stand." The goal of this message was to provide the basic information to family, friends, and acquaintances. I sent it to about forty people. As diagnoses, tests, and treatments continued, I wrote and emailed five more lengthy "where things stand" essays. Return emails invariably included requests for more facts and details as well as questions about the feelings I was experiencing. The final "where things stand" email that I sent after my radiation treatment was completed went to more than eighty people.

I was the one who benefited most from the "where things stand" emails. The act of writing was remarkably therapeutic, helping me internalize, understand, and articulate what was happening to me. Writing, and then editing, these emails was how I processed the complex information about my cancer and its treatment. One example: Writing these essays required fairly extensive research into how and why I could have an aggressive cancer with consistently "normal" PSA levels. But above all, the writing process kept Susan and me connected to people who cared deeply about what was happening to the two of us. Knowing that others were thinking about us and praying for us was a gift beyond words. Email is often derided as a coldly artificial means of communication. But in these circumstances, it was immensely comforting to know that upward of a hundred men and women who cared deeply formed a vital human connection. It's a cliché because it's true: Cancer is not something to be experienced in isolation, and communication technology can lessen that feeling of isolation that can so swiftly overtake us.

STIMULUS AND RESPONSE

Relationship experts tell us that effective communication must be a two-way street. This is especially true when cancer is the subject. As I noted earlier, the preexisting connections of "cancer" and "dread" in many people's minds often cause them to imagine only the worst possible outcome. Each individual responds differently when told by someone, "I have cancer," although most people will want to be positive. While it may seem selfish, I hoped people would respond to my news in supportive ways. That's why I tended to obsess over crafting the appropriate message for each target audience, using the same care I had devoted to my professional years of writing reports, product specifications, technical articles, press releases, and brochure copy. This required me to write and edit multiple drafts of each email, which in turn made me reflect more thoughtfully about the physical, psychological, and spiritual aspects of what was happening to Susan and me.

At least this was the theory. These experiments in communication did not always produce the responses I had anticipated. (And of course in some cases, there was no response at all.) The actual process of telling friends and family produced a panoply of reactions: some predictable, others less so. Susan and I told our adult children Geoff and Elisabeth first. Since they both live a long distance from our home in California, a phone call had to suffice. I briefly outlined the course of events leading up to Dr. Hopkins's succinct summary, "You have a nasty cancer." Their reactions were similar, yet each reflected their respective personalities. Both of them responded first with stunned disbelief, followed quickly by questions that revealed deep concern and caring. Geoff, a professor of philosophy, was thankfully not philosophical. Instead, he asked many factual questions, each reflecting his desire to deal with this news rationally, while maximizing information content. "What was the nature of the test?" "How do they know definitively that this is cancer?" "What is the next step to be taken?" "What can I do to help you both right now?" His tone was a mix of genuine sympathy and clear-eyed objectivity, which, given the emotion of the moment, was a much-needed elixir.

Elisabeth responded compassionately, and we could hear the tears in her voice over the speakerphone. "I wish I could be there with you and we could cry together," she said. She also asked detailed questions about how the cancer was discovered and what was coming next. We ended the conversation with her announcement that she would be coming to visit soon, but that right now she needed to seek out her friends for comfort.

Next, I told one of my closest friends Nancy, herself a cancer survivor. Once she and her husband recovered from their surprise, she offered a melancholy welcome to the club, a club, of course, that neither of us had wanted to join. Two months earlier she had completed an extensive course of chemotherapy treating a second bout of aggressive breast cancer that had surfaced after a twenty-year hiatus. Over dinner she advised, "Take it one day at a time. You'll want to remain flexible and avoid 'shoulds,' as in 'you really should complete that job,' or 'you should go see that person.'" Then she added, "The other thing not to forget: naps."

In talking about avoiding the "shoulds," Nancy addressed one of the key lessons I've learned in the months since the diagnosis: Cancer is sufficient unto itself; people with cancer are not required to prove anything to other people. Maintaining a clear boundary between who I am, and the expectations (especially the unspoken ones) of other people about my role as a "person with cancer" was essential. Otherwise, it was just too easy to slip noiselessly into the role of "cancer victim."

Of course, there were other people who were not cancer survivors who responded empathetically. I was—and remain—grateful to the numerous men and women who simply said, "I'll be praying for you." A number of them asked, "What can I do to help?" It was useful to be prepared with a short list of specific tasks people could do, such as "We would like to 'hang out' at your house for an afternoon between doctor appointments."

Even better were the people who said, "I want to help, and here's what I'd like to do." One of these people who came to us with a plan rather than a plaintive question was Karen, who brought meals to Susan and me—a godsend when I arrived home after radiation without energy or motivation to go near the kitchen. Another friend, Tom, drove me to several radiation treatment sessions, providing a break from the 5-day-a-week grind of a 52-mile round trip commute, as well as the opportunity to talk about topics completely unrelated to prostate cancer. Others sent cards, notes, and emails—each a boost to my spirits. The value of being surrounded by a caring community while being treated for cancer cannot be overstated.

DEALING WITH RESPONSES YOU WISH YOU HADN'T HEARD

Scattered among the hundreds of thoughtful and caring responses I received from my family, friends, and colleagues, there were a few reactions that were difficult to handle. For those who associated dread with cancer, their dread did not enhance their empathetic listening skills. The negative impact of hearing "I have cancer" from a family member or friend is probably second only to hearing "You have cancer" from one's own doctor. Yvonne Hanson compared the impact of hearing about a friend's cancer to that of hearing of a friend's death. American culture does an effective job of keeping death hidden from public view; until the past few years it has been almost as successful at hiding cancer. Many people wishing to discuss neither death nor cancer invariably deal with both euphemistically. I'm sure that in their hearts these people want to respond sympathetically, but they are compelled to do so without actually uttering the word "cancer." They may consent reluctantly to talking about the immediate situation, but will never broach the reality that the cancer may present life-threatening possibilities down the road. After listening to several people attempt to say the right thing while assiduously avoiding the idea of cancer itself, I sorted their deflective responses to my bad news into one of three categories: "jumpers," "minimizers," and "fixers."

A jumper's favorite expression is, "Don't worry. Everything will turn out fine." Variations included, "Every cloud has a silver lining," and worst of all, "God gives you only what you can handle. I know you'll be able to handle this." While responses like these were meant to be encouraging, in the end they felt like

Jumpers, Minimizers, and Fixers

Upon hearing the news of the diagnosis, the "jumpers" tended to rush immediately to the inevitably positive outcome they were convinced would occur, skipping right over any intervening unpleasantness that might be involved. Without actually saying so directly, the "minimizers" invariably made the point, usually unconsciously, that prostate cancer really wasn't a very big deal, subtly implying a person is exaggerating the gravity of their disease. The "fixers," on the other hand, invariably had specific advice about what you should do, whom you should see, or what treatment method you should embrace.

clichés that moved immediately to a happy ending—and jumped right over my need to process, and eventually to accept, the fact that aggressive cancer had become a reality in my life.

Following my diagnosis, I knew that numerous tests, procedures, and treatments lay ahead of me—and that many of them would be unpleasant. From my point of view, it would be a fairly long time (if ever) before I would be able to say, "Yes, indeed, everything did indeed turn out just fine." By focusing only on the happy ending, the jumpers inadvertently excluded the intermediate struggles that lay between now and then. These people essentially told me, "We really don't want to know the details. They really don't matter anyway since you know everything will be fine in the end." In my darker moments, whenever I heard a sentence starting or ending with "everything will turn out fine," I finished it in my mind, thinking, "… and you really don't want me to bore you with the details in the meantime, do you?"

Eventually, I decided that the "jumpers," by automatically presuming an optimistic outcome, did so because they were simply emotionally unable to entertain bad endings. My standard reply to their presumed sunny outcome became, "Well, I certainly hope so."

At least the "jumpers" always assumed a positive end point. I was less sure about the "minimizers." To be sure, prostate cancer has one of the highest cure rates of any cancer. But as I was looking down the long dark corridor of tests, procedures, and eventually, treatment, all these positive statistics missed the point of my individual experience with aggressive cancer. Rather than encouraging me, the minimizers only tended to deepen my gloom when they made comments like, "Oh, my husband had prostate cancer. They took it out and he's fine now." Or, "Prostate cancer has a high cure rate, you know." Yes, I already knew. Or, "My brother-in-law came through the surgery with flying colors. You'd never know he had cancer." Or, "Lance Armstrong beat cancer, and this year he's in the Tour de France." Well, I certainly hoped I'd have a great outcome, too, but I always felt their attempt to encourage me by the happy example of others trivialized the reality of my personal experience of this "common" cancer. "Prostate cancer just doesn't have the respect that those other cancers have," I grumbled inwardly, knowing that each individual's cancer is unique and will follow its own path. "Just because other people have had a nice outcome doesn't guarantee one for me."

Like the jumpers, the minimizers were signaling, again unintentionally, that they really couldn't listen to the details of my story. Despite their undeniable good intentions, their response always made me assume that they were thinking, "A lot of other men have survived prostate cancer. What do you think is so special about you?"

"Yes, you're right," I would think. "Prostate cancer is indeed common, and I'm certainly not the first one to have it. But at the same time, it's something unexpected, extraordinary, and scary that is happening to me—and all I really want is for you to acknowledge that." The minimizers' focus on what had happened to other people conspired to diminish my own experience, possibly even implying that I was just a whiner at heart. In the end, my response to the minimizers was simply to say, "I'm really glad things worked out well for him."

Many married men have probably heard their wives accuse them of trying to "fix" a problem rather than taking the time to listen sympathetically to their feelings. I certainly count myself among that oblivious multitude. But it was only after hearing several men tell me what I should do in order to cure my cancer did I really "get" what Susan had been telling me all these years about prescribing a quick fix without actually listening to her. "Fixer" statements I heard included:

- "You should go to Loma Linda and have the proton beam treatment."
- "Make sure you insist on robotic surgery."
- "I know a great urologist down at Stanford."

All these solutions were offered before I even had a definitive staging of my cancer, much less even knew what treatment options would be feasible for me. As with the jumpers and minimizers, these statements were made with a sincere intention to be helpful. But every fixer definitely hews to the cliché "Fire, ready, aim." Once again, all I could do was smile appreciatively and say, "That might be an option. We'll have to see how things go."

Within a few weeks of my diagnosis, I had pretty much gotten used to the jumpers, minimizers, and fixers. I always wanted to keep in mind that their intentions were harmless. Their messages were just clumsy. And, to be sympathetic to their good intentions, I would do well to remember that just as I had shocked Susan that morning I found out I had cancer, each well-wisher was dealing with his or her own form of shock as well. After all, they were hearing bad news from someone who they had always seen as being healthy and in control. Perhaps their reactions were simply another example of how cancer induces dread. It's even possible that my news forced them to examine their own mortality when they were unprepared to do so. They truly wanted to be helpful, but instead, they ended up jumping, minimizing, or fixing. I would do well to give them the benefit of the doubt. I had certainly responded in a similar manner to other people's problems at one time or another without realizing I might be doing harm.

By focusing on the caring intentions that lay behind their words, I could see they meant only the best for me. As time went on and they recovered from the initial shock, most of the jumpers, minimizers, and fixers eventually became sympathetic—even empathetic—listeners. Had I made the sarcastic responses that so greatly tempted me when I heard their comments, I would have hurt both them and me. In this instance, I was glad that I had chosen to be patient.

SIX

Full Speed Ahead

BUT FIRST, A CHANGE IN DIRECTION

One morning the phone rang as I walked into my office. The caller identified herself as Dr. Hopkins's assistant. Once she was assured that I was indeed Craig Pynn, she said, "The doctor would like to speak with you now." (This procedure has always irritated me since it sends such a clear message, whether intentionally or not, about whose time is considered more valuable.)

"Hi, Craig," Dr. Hopkins began. "Dr. Massullo and I have been talking about you. We've decided that we need to put you on androgen deprivation therapy (ADT) instead of the anti-androgen drugs you've been taking up to now."

"Uh, I thought you wanted to keep me on the anti-androgen because it has fewer side effects," I responded in surprise.

"I know there are more significant side effects with the ADT, but Dr. Massullo and I really feel this is the best approach in your case. We can talk about it more when you come in to have the gold balls inserted in a week or so. We'll also schedule a time for you to come in and get the ADT implant."

He concluded the call with the usual pleasantries. At first I was surprised, but I quickly became upset, since it was

Dr. Hopkins himself that had painted such a bleak picture of ADT's many side effects. He had described weight gain, bone and muscle mass loss, and loss of sexual function, making the ostensible cure for my cancer sound worse than the disease itself. By comparison, the anti-androgen therapy with its milder side effect of breast tenderness had been a far more attractive option. And my experience on the anti-androgen had indeed produced only some breast growth (gynecomastia). And now Dr. Hopkins suddenly decided to start me down what I understood to be the riskier ADT path.

For the first time in my relationship with my trusted urologist, I felt the need for a second opinion. My initial concern after hanging up the phone was that the doctors had some new data about my cancer that meant I needed the more aggressive ADT treatment. "What aren't they telling me?" I wondered darkly. The phone rang again, interrupting my train of thought. The caller ID read John Muir Radiation Oncology. This time there was no receptionist asking if I was Craig Pynn.

"Hi, Craig," Dr. Massullo said, "I called to tell you that Dr. Hopkins and I feel we need to move you over to androgen deprivation therapy before we start radiation." In the milliseconds before I answered him, I wondered if the two doctors had pre-arranged these two calls to reinforce their point.

"Yes, I just spoke with Dr. Hopkins," I answered. "Why is this change in direction necessary?" I asked. "When we started all this, Dr. Hopkins had said I'd be able to stay on the anti-androgen throughout the course of radiation."

"Well, the simple fact of the matter is that radiation plus ADT is the standard course for cancers like yours. There have been studies that demonstrate a definite therapeutic benefit of the two in combination. Radiation together with anti-androgen drugs is not practiced widely, if at all. And there has not yet been a study or any demonstrated benefit of using that combination.

"I admit that there are definitely more side effects with ADT, but we both think it's better to go with what we know," he concluded.

"Well, OK, I suppose, but this is certainly a surprise," I responded weakly. Once again, I had been caught off guard. In my state of mild shock, I could not even formulate any more detailed questions.

Hanging up, I felt both mild anxiety and weary resignation. My anxiety came from understanding the side effects of ADT treatment. Just two months ago, Dr. Hopkins had been quite unequivocal in our discussion about why he wanted me to take the anti-androgen rather than start ADT. In order to make his case for the anti-androgen, he had described in detail the numerous downsides of life in a body without testosterone. My subsequent Internet research had not only confirmed his point, but also revealed other negative side effects of the treatment, including hot flashes and loss of libido.

This far into the game, I felt as though the decision had already been made for me. Both doctors asserted there was really no sensible alternative to ADT if I planned to undertake the course of radiotherapy. And I later read at the National Cancer Institute (NCI) website (cancer.gov) that the combination of radiation and ADT had better "overall survival" outcomes than just radiation alone. Nevertheless, this was a sharp, unexpected turn in the tracks of the Oncology Adventure Ride. "Trust us," the doctors had implied, without actually uttering those words. A sense of resignation slowly edged out my anxiety, as I realized I'd joined a sizable, if not particularly cheerful, army of men who had already been down the same radiation and ADT road. They had survived, and I supposed I would, too.

This might have been a good time to seek a second opinion, but at this point, I just wanted to get on with it. "I'm sick of tests, procedures, and doctors, and there's much more to come," I whined inwardly. All those books and articles that focused on the clinical aspects of prostate cancer ignored this part, the emotional toll, when they advised getting second and even third and fourth opinions. This advice is easy to give when you are the author dispassionately writing a book. It's not so easy if you're the patient who must live with the physical and emotional consequences of the choice. The Oncology Adventure Ride, replete as it is with tests, discussions, procedures, and decisions—not to mention the treatments themselves—is exhausting. The cancer itself is exhausting. Enduring the medical decision-making process only amplifies this fatigue. When there was a sharp change of direction such as the one I had just experienced, the best I could do was just to hang on tight.

However, hanging on didn't mean accepting my fate without some knowledge and reassurance. I may have lacked the will and energy to seek out a second opinion from another doctor, but there were other ways to obtain fresh and varying points of view. The traditional method for obtaining a second opinion is to get the name of another doctor in the same field—often from the doctor giving the first opinion. Then, there's the bureaucratic process of obtaining insurance company approval, followed by securing the new doctor's agreement to provide the second opinion. Then, after the records are faxed over, there's the logistical exercise of arranging a consultation. I wondered how other men in my position had summoned the energy to execute all these steps. This cumbersome process may have worked well when information was scarce and almost always the exclusive property of the medical community. For me, anyway, getting a second opinion in the traditional manner seemed like using a rotary-dial telephone. The strategy would work, but it seemed to me that a simpler, more powerful technology was readily available, albeit one that needed to be used with caution.

THE INTERNET AS CANCER RESEARCH TOOL

Following my diagnosis, I had relied on the Internet to learn the basics of prostate cancer, so it was reasonable to expect there would be reliable information about the benefits of radiation combined with ADT compared to radiation combined with anti-androgen drugs. It didn't take long to find the details by searching on the phrase "radiation anti-androgen." The first item listed was a 2005 press release stating that a particular anti-androgen drug combined with radiation "extends life more than radiotherapy alone." But this document was light on details and failed to compare these results with the more traditional combination of ADT therapy and radiation. In fact, it didn't even mention ADT, which seemed like a significant omission, given that radiation plus ADT is the so-called "gold standard" or "standard of care" for locally advanced prostate cancer. Also, the press release emanated from the anti-androgen drug manufacturer itself, which undermined its credibility for me. I needed the most impartial information I could find.

I decided to go back to the two websites that had already provided reliable and objective information: The American Cancer Society ([ACS] www.cancer.org) and the National Cancer Institute ([NCI] www.cancer.gov). The NCI website is probably the most authoritative place on the web to find up-to-date technical information, especially about clinical trials. The prostate cancer area of the site features sections labeled "Health Professional Version" and "Patient Version." I certainly didn't qualify as a "Health Professional," but I figured I could wade through the arcane terminology and at least understand the gist of the articles. On the page describing clinical trial outcomes of various combinations of ADT, anti-androgen, and radiation, I hit the informational jackpot. The most pertinent section about ADT plus external beam radiotherapy directly substantiated what Dr. Massullo had asserted during our phone call:

> *Randomized clinical trial evidence comparing radiation therapy to radiation therapy with prolonged androgen suppression ... was evaluated. The meta-analysis found a difference in 5-year OS [overall survival] in favor of radiation therapy plus continued androgen suppression compared with radiation therapy alone.*

So, these researchers were saying that androgen suppression, meaning ADT, combined with radiation produced the best outcome in terms of survival. The verdict for treatment with an anti-androgen drug plus radiotherapy was rendered farther down on the same page:

> *[The anti-androgen drug] has not been shown to improve OS in patients with localized or locally advanced prostate cancer. [An] international trial compared [the anti-androgen drug] (150 mg orally per day) plus standard care (radical prostatectomy, radiation therapy, or watchful waiting, depending on local custom) with standard care alone for men with nonmetastatic localized or locally advanced prostate cancer. [...] At a median follow-up of 7.4 years, there was no difference in OS between [the anti-androgen drug] and placebo groups.*

This research-speak basically said that the anti-androgen drug had no discernable effect on extending the lives of men with advanced prostate cancer. As far as I was concerned, this was the informational equivalent to a second opinion, especially since the results of my urethral biopsy had definitively diagnosed my cancer as being locally advanced. The range of effective treatment options for my case was therefore limited. For my particular circumstances, the best treatment option did indeed seem to be the one recommended by my two doctors. Not everyone would agree with—nor should they necessarily follow—my approach of seeking out reliable data on the Internet to confirm what my urologist and radiation oncologist had recommended, especially those who prefer human opinions to information contained in journal articles. Granted, research performed by the patient himself carries risks, but reliable resources such as the NCI site have made this approach easier and less risky in recent years.

The Internet has greatly leveled the informational playing field. Now, at a minimum, the abstracts of virtually every journal article from the last ten years are available online at the extensive PubMed article database maintained by the National Center for Biotechnology Information. In many cases, the complete articles themselves are also available. Locating, reading, and interpreting technical papers and articles that described my situation went a long way toward alleviating my lack of knowledge about the disease inside me. Access to information also reduced my feeling that others—albeit experienced professionals—were dictating my fate. I never doubted that my doctors had my best interests at heart and that their recommendations were based on their years of experience and practiced skill. But being able to confirm independently what they had told me increased my confidence in the course they wanted me to follow. Being able to accomplish this on the Internet—rather than having to test my doctors against the opinion of some unknown third doctor—also eased my anxiety, not to mention saving significant time and energy. Best of all, even with this unexpected change in direction on the Oncology Adventure Ride, I felt much more confident and ready to get on with treatment itself.

To be fair, I should explain that my experience does not mean that the Internet is always a reliable substitute for a qualified second opinion. Even though prostate cancer is an all-too-ordinary disease, every man's case is unique. My situation was exceptional because the urethral biopsy had proved that my cancer had spread beyond the confines of the prostate gland, thereby narrowing the scope of treatment options. Further, as we have all been repeatedly warned, the Internet must be used cautiously and judiciously. It certainly offers rapid access to a vast repository of information, but the quality and validity of that information ranges widely in its credibility. Just as a reporter needs to know and trust his or her sources, the Internet researcher must be ruthlessly discriminating. There is a big difference between self-serving press releases issued by companies marketing their pharmaceutical products and clinical trial data from the National Cancer Institute. However, used carefully, Internet-based information is by far the most efficient way to become a better-informed patient with a modest investment of time and effort.

So, after confirming the information online, I took a deep breath, called both doctors, and gave my assent for the course they recommended, radiation plus androgen deprivation therapy. Still, there were many steps to be navigated between my agreement and actually starting my treatment.

INSERTED, SIMULATED, IMPLANTED, AND INFUSED

Soon after my conversations with the doctors, an administrator from Pacific Urology called. "We need you to go the John Muir Radiation Oncology Department and pick up your gold seeds." These were the tiny gold spheres that would serve as the X-ray reference markers (sometimes called "fiducials") inside my prostate to further improve the accuracy of the X-rays that would be aimed at my prostate during radiotherapy. The voice continued, "Then, please drop them off here at our office. Dr. Hopkins can insert them next Monday." Her matter-of-fact tone made the process sound as routine as having a plumber come to install a new faucet.

"Uh, O.K.," I replied, shuddering a bit at the word "insert."

"Also," the administrator continued, "we're scheduling you to come in ten days to get your hormone implant." The phrase "hormone treatment (HT)" is the stand-in euphemism often used for ADT (even though the whole point of ADT is not to receive a hormone, but to eliminate one—specifically testosterone). "An hour after you receive the hormone implant, we'll give you an infusion of Zometa® for your osteopenia."

As I hung up the phone, I realized that my prostate cancer treatment course was now moving into high gear. Metaphorically, I could hear the clanking chain as the Oncology Adventure Ride slowly hauled me up to the highest part of the ride, poised to careen down through actual treatment. At this point, I imagined that the eight-and-a-half week ride through the Treatment Loop would be scary, frustrating, or exhilarating, or probably a mix of all three. Until the radiation treatments actually started, I was going to be an increasingly anxious and impatient cancer patient.

Returning to the Radiation Oncology Center the next day, I approached the receptionist's window and identified myself. "We expected you yesterday," the receptionist remarked amiably. "Here you go, Craig." She smiled as she handed me a flat, sealed plastic bag about four inches by twelve inches. Inside I could see four fierce-looking metal rods that looked like they fit into some sort of trigger-actuated instrument. The mechanism that came to mind was a small crossbow, and the rods resembled miniature arrows. At the end of the arrow tips were the barely visible gold "seeds" that would end up permanently lodged in my prostate. After transporting the package two miles up the road, I left it with the receptionist at Pacific Urology.

The following Monday afternoon, I was back at Pacific Urology in the same exam room where the fateful prostate biopsy had occurred three months before. "I know the routine," I told Dr. Hopkins's assistant and began undressing as she exited the room. Naked from the waist down, I assumed my position on my left side on the narrow exam table. Minutes later, Dr. Hopkins walked in, smiled warmly, and shook my hand, even as I lay awkward and exposed. After receiving a numbing shot of lidocane, the doctor placed one of the gold-tipped arrows into something that looked like a spring-loaded caulking gun, only smaller. We chatted as he found the correct prostatic location using his ultrasound probe, inserted the gun up my rectum, and pulled the trigger of the device that inserted the gold seed. Numbed by the lidocaine, I felt only a slight bump. This procedure was certainly less painful than the biopsy.

"I'm really happy about your prostate; it looks almost normal," he exclaimed.

"Cool," I grunted. At least making conversation distracted me from what else was happening at the moment.

"I'm really very pleased with how well the anti-androgen has shrunk your prostate. Be sure to tell Dr. Massullo that it really was extremely enlarged before. He may not believe me."

"Sure," I replied. "Maybe it was someone else's enlarged prostate you were thinking of; mine's actually normal; and we really don't have to go through this whole radiation business." He responded with a laugh, clearly indicating that we were definitely still going ahead with the radiation treatments.

Since there were only four gold seeds, the insertion process was relatively quick. After I dressed, Dr. Hopkins showed me the MRI scan I had had a few weeks earlier. Pointing to an indistinct blob in the center of my urological anatomy, he said "This darker area may represent an 'irregularity.' But I don't see anything extraordinary. Contrary to some claims, prostate cancer really doesn't image very well, and it's rarely visible on a standard CT or MRI scan."

I briefly summarized my meeting with Dr. Massullo, mentioning that he had shown me the Memorial Sloan-Kettering nomograms that indicated I had a 93 percent probability of surviving five years.

"Well, those are the statistics, but your particular case is out of the box." The unspoken implication was glaringly clear: "Don't get your hopes up so high, buddy. Those statistics may not apply to you."

That afternoon I went home and wrote an optimistic "where things stand" email for my friends, calculating that at the then-current price of gold ($942.00 per ounce), each 8 cubic millimeter gold sphere in my prostate was worth about $50, increasing the net worth of my body by about two hundred dollars. As the price of gold fluctuates over the remainder of my life, so, too, will my body's monetary value.

The "where things stand" email I sent that day was more upbeat than the earlier ones. I received many cheery replies in turn, congratulating me on the good news. I could sense the relief in people's replies; suggesting that a number of my correspondents believed I was pretty much cured at this point. This made me feel better, even though I hadn't even started radiation yet. Then again, I hadn't told anyone about Dr. Hopkins's comment that my case was "out of the box." I kept that particular worry to myself.

That evening I wrote in my journal:

> *So, this is the "Big C." What should it be doing to my feelings? I'm not really sure. Right now, I feel the course I'm on is pretty curative and barring other (non-cancer) events, I should be around for a fairly long time. Although not as long as I once assumed. I'm pretty sure that my life expectancy has been shortened by my cancer. Strangely, I feel very little anxiety about that—except sometimes when I wake up in the middle of the night. There are some very good reasons for my equanimity: Susan, our children, their spouses, and close friends at Saint Matthew [our church] offering prayers and encouragement.*

As it turned out, my optimism proved somewhat premature.

Ten days after I had the gold balls inserted, I was back the "Rad Onc" lab. After only a short wait, the technician bounced into the waiting room with a smile and outstretched hand. "Hi, Craig. I'm Shari. I'm one of the radiation techs here, and I'll be doing your simulation. Let me show you where to change."

Shari was short, blonde, and attractive. Her infectious smile seemed to come from a deeper place than the somewhat artificial cheerfulness I had often encountered from other clinicians. As I came to know her and the other radiation technicians over the coming weeks, it was clear that they took their jobs seriously, but they could also inject some levity into the proceedings. I think it requires a special empathy to maintain heartfelt good humor in the face of unrelenting, mostly cancer-ridden woe, and I came to greatly admire the entire staff at Rad Onc. Of course, I never forgot that it was their collective skill on which survival depended.

In the locker room, I donned what would become my "radiation uniform" for the next two and a half months: hospital-issue pajama bottoms, socks, and the polo shirt I was wearing when I walked into the lab. Shari was standing in the patient's waiting area when I emerged. She silently led me to the simulation lab.

At the center of the room stood a standard issue Siemens CT scan X-ray machine. "Lie down right here," she said, pointing to the hard, narrow table covered with a folded white sheet. The table, mounted atop a sliding mechanism, stood out in front of the doughnut-hole-shaped opening of the CT scanner. This tabletop ride on its straight, short tracks guiding me through the scanner opening looked much less exciting than the one on my metaphorical roller coaster. Shari placed a triangular piece of stiff foam under my knees and a small foam block under my head. In the coming weeks I would come to appreciate the small comfort afforded by these stiff pieces of medical foam, as they greatly reduced the rigid table's discomfort on my lower back. I was pretty content, except for the full bladder I'd been instructed to arrive with—a standing requirement for prostate radiation treatments that had not been mentioned on any of the websites about radiotherapy that I had visited.

Looking up at the ceiling I spied the red lasers: one mounted on the ceiling directly above me, another on the wall in front of me, and two more, one on each of the walls to the side of the machine. These lasers mounted on the walls and ceiling separate radiation oncology equipment from ordinary X-ray and CT scan machines. They are essential to the all-important calibration task, making sure the radiation beam is directed to the proper location in the patient's body. Slightly tilting my head up from the table, I could see the lasers' thin red lines bisecting my body from three different directions.

Shari untied my pajama bottoms and pulled them down a few inches. I should have expected this. Where prostate issues are concerned, preserving modesty is impossible. To the doctors and technicians, I was just another male body. Shari used a small control box dangling on a cord from the ceiling to shift the table into the proper position.

"OK, we've got you where we want you," she said, a remark that seemed to have several levels of meaning. She then picked up a black Sharpie® laundry marker and drew three black crosses on my body. She had drawn each cross squarely at the intersection of each of the red laser lines that traced across my body: one cross on each hip and the third squarely in the middle of my pubic area. As she covered each black cross with transparent waterproof tape, she said, "Now, you need to make sure these crosses stay visible on your body for the next two weeks, since they mark the alignment locations that we'll be using for the actual radiation treatments. If they start to wear off, just come into the lab and we'll happily re-mark them for you. Now, we're going image your pelvic area so the physicist can develop your actual radiation plan. Be sure to lie completely still." She left the room, and the CT scanner whirred to life. My bladder felt extraordinarily full at this point, and it was difficult to comply with Shari's order to remain motionless. Finally the scan ended, and she reappeared.

"That's it. We'll see you in two weeks." Happily, there was a restroom right across the hall.

That night as I stood naked in front of the bathroom mirror, I could see the three crosses, each with a black circle drawn around them. "Well, it is Lent," I thought. "The three crosses are definitely a symbolic kind of Lenten discipline."

The preparation for radiotherapy was moving quickly now. Just two weeks remained until my first session. The day after my simulation, I was once again at Pacific Urology, where by now, the receptionists knew both my first and last name. This visit was for an implant and an infusion. Someone had apparently modified the schedule, and the receptionist informed me that I was going to have both procedures at the same time. "Great," I mused, feeling ironic. "Minor surgery and an IV simultaneously. How lucky can I get?"

The androgen deprivation drugs that were to turn off testosterone production are termed luteinizing hormone-releasing hormone (LHRH) agonists. The drug mimics the action of the naturally occurring LHRH hormone generated in the brain's hypothalamus by binding to receptors in the pituitary gland—occupying the parking spaces for the natural LHRH, as it were. Since the natural LHRH cannot attach to its receptors the pituitary cannot send its chemical message to the testes—where 95 percent of a man's testosterone is manufactured—to produce the male hormone. The urologist can choose from a wide variety of LHRH agonist drugs. The most widely used drug, Lupron®, is administered by injection, usually every three months. Dr. Hopkins had already decided that I needed to remain testosterone-free for at least two years—probably more. Accordingly, he chose a relatively new drug packaged as a small plastic implant that provided a one-year supply of the LHRH agonist. It would reside in my left bicep for a year before being dug out and replaced with a new implant for my second year of ADT.

By contrast, Zometa® (zoledronic acid) was infused via a standard IV. Originally, zoledronic acid was developed to strengthen bone in order to prevent skeletal fractures in cancer patients. Since it can help prevent osteoporosis, it is also widely marketed and administered to post-menopausal women. In my case, the purpose of the zoledronic acid was to strengthen my bones, since a prominent side effect of androgen deprivation therapy is loss of bone mass. Because I was already predisposed to osteoporosis, Dr. Hopkins viewed this infusion every three months as an essential countermeasure to the bone-weakening effects of living without testosterone.

On this visit I was led to an unfamiliar exam room. Dr. Hopkins's assistant appeared, pushed a metal table up on my left side, placing my forearm on the table as I tried to shift to a more comfortable position. Alongside my arm, I saw gauze, a syringe, and multiple sterile instruments, including what looked like a scalpel. The assistant left the room. Moments later a pleasant, fiftyish woman appeared and introduced herself. "Hi, I'm Elizabeth, Dr. Hopkins's nurse. I'm here to give you the infusion."

"This feels like stereo," I quipped, using an inappropriate metaphor. "Left arm for implant; right for infusion. By the way, the last time someone tried to give me an IV it took four tries," I added nervously.

"That won't be a problem," she said, immediately proving her skill by sticking the IV in a vein in the back of my right hand on the first try.

"Nice work," I replied gratefully. We chatted about various non-medical topics as the bag of Zometa and saline solution slowly emptied its contents into my arm. The bag was about half empty when Dr. Hopkins entered the room.

"Sorry I'm late," he apologized. "I had a consult on a particularly tough case, and you never know just how long these things will take." This seemed like the perfect invitation to test something that my friend Chuck had told me recently. He said that if you have to have cancer you want to be a cancer case that's boring to the doctors because it's so familiar that they know exactly what to do. "Happily, I was a boring case," Chuck had said about himself.

"So, Doc, then you must be glad to see me since I'm a pretty ordinary—even boring—case for you," I said as casually as I could.

"Well, not really," Hopkins replied as he applied a syringe of local anesthetic to my bicep. "You have extensive cancer."

Hearing those four words felt almost as devastating as hearing the original scary words, "You have a nasty prostate cancer," two months before. Logically, I shouldn't have been surprised. From the information I had from my previous doctors' visits combined with what I had learned via the Internet, I knew that the fact that my cancer had migrated to my urethra was highly unusual, as was the fact that I had the unhappy combination of a low PSA and an aggressive tumor. Chuck's colorectal cancer may have been a boring case, but mine wasn't a boring case of prostate cancer. In the words of the famous TV philosopher, Fred Rogers, I was—even if I did not want to be—"special."

I looked away as the doctor lifted the scalpel. I felt some pushing and shoving, but happily no pain. In a few minutes he announced the drug was in and the incision sutured. Now injected, simulated, implanted, and infused, I was finally ready for my course of radiotherapy.

I CRIED TODAY

My repeated wanderings between Pacific Urology, Rad Onc, and the medical lab near my home for blood tests, imaging studies, and scans had finally come to a temporary end. Suddenly—medically speaking, at least—there was only silence. Still, I was a week away from my first radiotherapy session. Without the distractions of doctors, nurses, techs, and tests, I could finally reflect on my situation. I was a locally advanced prostate cancer patient with what my doctor termed an "out of the box" extensive cancer. After so many months of focusing my efforts on understanding the physical events that were happening inside my body, a deep, searing anger at my predicament finally surfaced. My uninvited dance partner had been holding me in a suffocating embrace for months, and I now, realized it had no intention of letting go.

One warm California day, early enough in the spring that the hillsides were still covered with lush green grass and yellow mustard, Susan and I decided to take what started out as a carefree drive. Later that afternoon, after we had returned home in angry silence, I wrote in my journal:

I cried today. I haven't cried for many, many years. Not like this. These were not the teary eyes that movies and heartwarming stories can sometimes induce. But curled-up-on-the-bed sobs and tears running down my face. And deep, deep overwhelming sadness.

The day had begun so well. Susan and I had a delightful ride through the green Contra Costa hills and a delicious lunch at our favorite restaurant on San Francisco Bay, sitting, talking and admiring the fog as it crept through the Golden Gate, across the Marin hills and the Bay itself.

Driving home along the Eastshore Freeway in Berkeley I expressed my impatience at a slow driver in the left lane, abruptly cutting her off. Not once but twice. The action was hostile, and it was clearly my fault. And then came the silence: her silence, my silence. Both of us were looking straight ahead at the road, interrupted by occasional sidelong glances at each other. I knew she was angry with me. That in turn made me angry with her. For the next few miles I engaged in some "that-driver-shouldn't-have-been-slow-poking-in-the-left-lane" rationalization while Susan sighed with some long-suffering "it's-all-my-fault-because-you're-always-right" statements by her. Followed by more silence—all the way home.

Yes, I guess I feel sorry for myself. And I shouldn't, I know. But...

> *I'm tired of being the Good Son.*
> *I'm tired of being the Good Christian.*
> *I'm tired of being the Good Husband.*
> *And now, above all else, I'm tired of being the Good Cancer Patient.*

I resent that the hormone that defines my manhood is being taken away from me for the next two years and maybe more. I resent that some big machine, however accurately, is going to fry my insides for the next eight-and-a-half weeks.

I'm pissed that in so many ways this damned disease seems to have come to define who I am. Perhaps not by other people, but I think very much by me.

So, I lay on the bed and cried. Yes, I know I should probably be praying for patience instead. I should be grateful for the medical technology that will help heal me. I should be thankful for all the people around me—most especially Susan, who truly loves me and truly cares for me. I should ... I should ...

But who am I, if I am defined only by the "shoulds" in my life?

PART III

THE OTHER REALITIES OF PROSTATE CANCER

SEVEN

The Business of Cancer Treatment

TABLE FOR ONE

On a warm spring evening in early April—some two and a half months after being diagnosed—I recorded some thoughts in my journal. My first radiation session was scheduled for the following morning. "I feel a little nervous," I wrote. "Yes, I know intellectually that radiation is the optimal course for my particular cancer. But it all seems so unconvincing. It would have been nice to have had it cut out and be done with it." I envied my friend Denny who had been diagnosed with a clean, fully-contained-within-the-prostate tumor that was surgically excised by robotic prostatectomy. The radiation I was about to undergo seemed like a more complicated path to a cure. Not to mention a more inconvenient one—I was about to begin a daily fifty-two mile round trip commute to the Radiation Oncology Center for the next nine weeks. "On the other hand," I wrote, "there are no knives involved with radiation."

The next morning, I arrived fifteen minutes early and waved my newly issued radiation oncology photo ID under the barcode reader at the reception desk. My card swipe let the techs in the back know I had arrived. After changing into my radiation patient's uniform and sitting a few minutes in the small waiting area, the door opened.

"Your table for one is ready, Craig." A tall blond woman with a wide smile appeared. "Hi, I'm Gretchen. Come on back." I guessed this was not the first time she had used the "table for one" joke to relax a nervous first-time radiotherapy patient.

I followed her back, padding along in my stockinged feet as we passed a work area filled with computer monitors, looking like command central. We walked through a large, heavy-looking open door. It felt about ten degrees colder inside the treatment room. Before me stood a large, imposing machine: the Siemens Primus linear accelerator. The staff simply called it "the Primus." Standing about eight feet tall, sheathed in beige-painted sheet metal, its most noticeable feature was a large gantry designed to rotate the collimator—the part that emitted the actual radiation—360 degrees around the treatment table.

Many people mistakenly believe that linear accelerators used for radiotherapy produce radioactivity, when in fact they produce X-rays (or "radiation" for short) of sufficiently high power to damage the DNA of cancer cells so that they die ("apoptosis") when they attempt to reproduce. Healthy cells damaged by radiation can repair themselves. X-rays are comprised of photons, exactly the same packets of energy that make up visible light but only at much higher power levels and also at much higher frequencies than our eyes can detect. While the machines used for radiation therapy are large, they are simple in concept. A linear accelerator, a smaller version of the accelerators used in physics labs to generate and study sub-atomic particles, creates high-powered X-rays. This energy is directed by copper plumbing through the collimator head, which like the camera shutter it resembles, can be programmed to a variety of shapes. Along with its shape, the energy intensity of the beam is varied, or "modulated, by the treatment program to "paint" the radiation to conform to the shape of the tumor. The gantry rotates around the patient to perform this painting task from different directions.

My technical knowledge of the machine's operation did little to make the Primus less intimidating. The narrow treatment table stood a few feet in front of the gantry. It was about six feet in length and almost three feet off the ground. As I discovered shortly after I lay on it the first time, the table was elevated to about four and a half feet off the ground for the actual treatment—not a height from which you'd want to accidentally roll off. The table itself was jet black, made of a carbon composite of some sort and was partially covered by a folded white sheet. The same triangular foam block that I had used at the simulation two weeks earlier was in place, together with the smaller rectangular block for my head to rest on.

As we entered the treatment room, Gretchen asked me to place my ID card under another bar code reader. I saw the same photo as the one on my ID appear on the computer screen. "We just need to make sure we're treating the right person," Gretchen explained.

From behind me a softly accented voice said, "Just crawl up on the table." He was a thin middle-aged man with a broad smile. "Hi, Craig. I'm Renato."

"Great to meet you," I replied, carefully scooching into place on the table that was no more that twenty-four inches wide—and extremely hard. The formal term for the table is "patient couch," but its lack of cushioning made "table" the more appropriate term. I adjusted my body into position, as Renato untied my pajama bottoms, pulling them down while simultaneously pushing up my shirt up above my navel, then thoughtfully placed a white towel across my exposed parts.

There I lay unprotected, as if on some sacrificial altar awaiting the arrival of a knife-wielding Aztec priest. Renato slid the table closer to the back of the machine. The collimator head was now directly over my pelvis. I could see the three orthogonal beams tracing thin red lines across my body. As in the simulation room, these came from lasers mounted in the ceiling and three walls. Renato quickly aligned the still-visible black crosses with the red shafts of light.

"Now, lie perfectly still; don't try to help us as we adjust your position," Renato instructed. He stood on my right, Gretchen on my left. "OK, I need a tug," he said. Gretchen grabbed the edge of the sheet and, yes, tugged it, shifting my body about an inch to the left. "Now a roll," he said. I felt a smaller tug this time. As I found out later, "tug," "roll," and "nudge" each have a specific dimensional meaning when radiation techs are aligning the patient to the lasers.

Renato turned to me. "OK, today, we'll be X-raying you from all the directions we'll be using for the actual treatment. It will feel just like an actual radiation session, except that there'll be no radiation. We'll start treatment tomorrow." His announcement disappointed me: All this preparation leading up to the Big Moment, only to find out I was not yet there. I felt like I was at the very top of a roller coaster, at the moment when the car pauses momentarily, and I was staring straight down into the abyss just ahead. The momentary halt just heightened the anticipation—and the dread.

Renato was holding a green Sharpie marker in his hand. "We're going to draw an outline of the radiation field on your right hip and pubic area to make sure the machine is programmed correctly. Then we're going to take a photograph of the outlines and show it to the doctor." A light turned on somewhere inside the collimator, and an oddly shaped pattern of light appeared over my pubic area. Renato traced the irregular outline of the light in green Sharpie. Using a manual control to rotate the collimator 90 degrees so it was pointed at my right side, he traced a second, differently shaped outline on my hip. I asked Renato why he didn't mark on my left side. He replied that the treatment shape on right hip would be the mirror image of the left and that the same went for front and back. He then whipped out a small digital camera and took a couple of shots. I have always been grateful that I never saw those photographs.

When I examined my naked body in the mirror later that night, I saw the black crosses and the strangely shaped green outlines that delineated the radiation field. The area on my front was roughly rectangular, about 4 inches wide and 6 inches long. The marking on my hip was a jagged outline, about 5 inches by 6 inches. I was impressed by how precisely the medical professionals could shape the radiation field.

After Renato had completed taking the photos, he and Gretchen left the room. While I knew that people who work around X-rays always leave the room for their own protection, I couldn't help but reflect on the irony that the 6 million electron volts of X-ray energy that they were protecting themselves from was being aimed straight at my private parts. At least at the dentist's office they covered my chest with a lead apron while taking X-rays of my teeth—and those X-rays were much weaker by comparison. Here, only a white sheet separated me from their destructive power. The Primus was now my only companion in the room, a large, intimidating apparatus whose therapeutic value I had to take on faith. Even though it was sheathed in impressive technology, I knew that at its core it was designed to do one thing only: sauté my insides, albeit with exquisite accuracy, in order to damage the DNA of the cancer cells so they could not reproduce.

"The Oncology Adventure Ride has now entered the Prostate Cancer Industrial Zone," I mused. The machine came to life as the gantry began to rotate silently around my body.

THE PROSTATE CANCER TREATMENT MARKET

As a marketing professional, I habitually frame new experiences in the terminology of my craft, such as "What is the size of the total available market?" or "How does this product compete with similar, already available products?" These may seem like unusual thoughts to have running through one's head while lying on a treatment table in a radiation oncology center. When cancer is your dance partner, a person's focus would usually be on surviving the ordeal, not the size and characteristics of the cancer treatment market. Yet, as I lay there motionless under the Primus, contemplating its probable price tag, I realized that there were probably hundreds of prostate cancer patients around the United States at this same moment in the exact same position. That added up to a lot of expensive radiation equipment. Then I thought about how many other prostate cancer patients might be in surgery at that moment. Or how many of them were also taking the same expensive anti-androgen and androgen suppression drugs that I was. Clearly, there was serious money in the prostate cancer treatment business.

First, how big is the prostate cancer treatment market? After all, more than 200,000 men in the United States are diagnosed each year with prostate cancer, the most prevalent male cancer. That number is equivalent to a city the size of Rochester, New York. A new case is diagnosed about every two and a half minutes around the clock. About 2 million prostate cancer patients and survivors are alive today. And, sadly, more than 30,000 men die from the disease each year, making prostate cancer the second biggest cause of cancer-related deaths among American men, after lung cancer. A nonsmoking man is more likely to get prostate cancer than lung, bronchus, colon, rectal, bladder, lymphoma, melanoma, oral, and kidney cancers—combined.

These numbers are substantial enough to make prostate cancer treatment a significant and attractively profitable market to a variety of equipment and pharmaceutical suppliers—not to mention urologists and oncologists. And, as with all markets, it's important first to understand the characteristics of the consumers of these prostate cancer treatment options.

While prostate cancer is often relegated to the category of an "old man's disease"—67 is the median age at diagnosis—it certainly affects younger men, as well. In fact, slightly more than 40% of men diagnosed are under the age of 65. Since I was younger than average when I was diagnosed at 62 years old, the fact that I had become an unwilling member of what some thoughtlessly called an "old man's club" had not helped my psychological reaction to having this disease. But what, I wondered, are some of the other dimensions that define this market?

The National Cancer Institute tracks U.S. cancer statistics of all sorts—including mortality rates—in its Surveillance Epidemiology and End Results (SEER) database. The death rate due to prostate cancer, while lower than some other types of cancer, is unevenly distributed among races. In 2009, SEER estimated that, of one hundred thousand men in the general population, about twenty-six men die from prostate cancer each year. Whites die at a rate of 23.6 per hundred thousand. The death rate among Asians is 10.6 per hundred thousand, and among Hispanics, it is 19.6 deaths per hundred thousand. Among African Americans, however, the death rate is double that of whites, at 56.3 deaths per hundred thousand men per year.

Prostate Mortality Rates by Ethnicity

(Deaths per hundred thousand men in that population)

White	23.6
Asian	10.6
Hispanic	19.6
African American	56.3

Numerous studies have examined (and continue to examine) the reasons behind the African American disparity. There may be genetic factors that make African American men inherently more vulnerable to the disease. Also, while men of all races work hard to avoid doctor visits, Black men are even less likely to have their PSA tested because, as a group, they are underserved by the medical community in the United States. In the end, the root causes are probably a combination of these—and doubtless numerous other—biological and societal factors.

Another way to divide up the prostate cancer target market is by "stage distribution," which measures the progression of the cancer. SEER notes that about 80 percent of prostate cancer diagnoses are "local" (Stage I and Stage II, contained within the confines of the prostate gland itself), 12 percent are "regional" (Stage III, also termed "locally advanced"), and 4 percent are "distant" or metastasized (Stage IV). The remaining 3 percent are classified as "unknown staging."

As I tried to absorb these numbers, I reflected on how statistics so effectively mask the individual stories, experiences, and feelings of the individual men who make up these numbers. Behind the massive SEER database, consisting of hundreds of thousands of records, was an equal number of human beings that had heard the ugly sentence, "You have cancer." Not only had they heard it, but they also had had to deal with its physical, emotional, and spiritual consequences.

For every one hundred men diagnosed with prostate cancer, there were approximately twelve men like me with locally advanced cases where the tumor had already escaped the confines of the prostate gland when they were diagnosed. These men had also heard their doctors use phrases like "out of the box," "aggressive," "inoperable," and perhaps, "you should have come to see me sooner." I wondered how these other men, whom I would never meet but who were in the same situation as I was, were dealing with their own particular circumstances. I resolved not to forget them. Behind the numbers that comprised this "market," there were real individuals with a real disease, real feelings, and, too often, real fear.

Prostate tumors are generally (although not always) slow growing. With the help of PSA screening that came into widespread use in the US during the late 1980s, most prostate cancer is usually found at earlier stages than other types of cancers. Many men who are diagnosed with localized cancers may not actually require treatment—at least not in the near term. Early diagnosis and slow-growing tumors give prostate cancer patients high survival rates, especially for the 80 percent of men who are diagnosed with "local" Stage I or II cancer. Statistically, local cancers of the prostate have a 100 percent survival rate after five years. Locally advanced Stage III cancers like mine have survival rates at five years that are almost as good. However, at ten and fifteen years after diagnosis and treatment, survival rates of localized cancers still remain above 90 percent, while the survival rate for locally advanced cancers like mine decreases to 50 to 60 percent. By contrast, at five years out, only about 30 percent of men diagnosed with metastasized Stage IV prostate cancer will still be alive.

These are just a few of the dimensions of today's prostate cancer treatment market. As the baby boomer population ages and more men are diagnosed, the need for prostate cancer treatment will grow, as will the need for treatment of all types of cancer. Because of this aging population, total deaths from prostate cancer each year will also increase. A June 2009 article published in the *Journal of Clinical Oncology* notes, "One of the most defining socio-demographic changes ongoing in the United States is the dramatic increase in the number of older adults and minorities. Specifically, the number of adults age 65 or older increased from 25 million in 1980 to 35 million in 2000, and is further expected to increase to 72 million by 2030 as the baby boomer generation ages."

Using SEER data, the authors estimate that the number of diagnoses of cancers of all kinds will increase 45 percent from about 1.6 million in 2010 to 2.3 million in 2030. Prostate cancer will be a major contributor to this growth, with an estimated 55 percent increase from around 200,000 diagnosed cases in 2010 to 380,000 cases in 2030, the year by which the "trailing edge" baby boomers born in 1964 will have turned 65. The authors drily observe "the striking increase in cancer incidence and correspondingly an increase in cancer prevalence could exceed the capacity of the current health care system." More ominously, they claim that, "the increasing incidence of cancer, coupled with the rising cost to treat an individual cancer patient, could exert a synergistic effect on growth of cancer costs." In other words, the growing numbers of cancer patients multiplied by the growing cost to treat each patient is ultimately unsustainable. These numbers underlie the need for comprehensive reform of the American health care system based on rational analysis instead of political calculation.

But what is considered unsustainable expense on one side of the ledger is revenue—and profit—on the other side. For the practitioners and companies in the prostate cancer treatment business, these numerical predictions identify what some marketers (usually behind closed doors) call a "sweet spot": a target market that is increasing numerically, as well as generating growing revenue per customer as treatment costs continue to escalate.

For every disease there are three potential sources of revenue: prevention, diagnosis, and treatment. Despite extensive research, there is no one direct cause of prostate cancer such as the clear link between tobacco use and lung cancer. Prostate cancer's likely cause appears to be some mix of genetics, diet, overall physical health, and the environment—a mix that varies greatly in each individual case. Despite extensive research, no root cause has emerged, nor is one likely to emerge. As a result, prostate cancer prevention strategies remain elusive. Consequently, expenditures on prostate cancer prevention by either the government or insurance companies are miniscule given the prevalence of the disease in the U.S. population. Instead, prevention remains pretty much in the domain of diet gurus and practitioners of holistic medicine. Some revenue comes from diagnosis, but PSA testing and biopsies produce little income compared to the cash generated by actually treating prostate cancer.

Treatment is where the money is—and will continue to be. Even assuming that treating one case of prostate cancer costs a relatively modest ten thousand dollars, 200,000 annual diagnoses add up to a substantial sum. While market researchers disagree about the precise annual revenue, they agree that treating prostate cancer is a multi-billion dollar market, one that will only increase in step with the growing populations of minorities and aging baby boomers over the next twenty years.

Organizations ranging from local hospitals and urology practices to multi-national pharmaceutical companies are eagerly participating—or planning to participate—in treating the hundreds of thousands of men diagnosed with prostate cancer each year. Of course, this business model could change in unexpected ways because of recent health care reform legislation. It's impossible to predict what kind of impact reform may have for prostate cancer's many different treatment methods, and therefore for its different market segments. One thing is sure: Treatment providers will always follow the money. Regardless of government policy or insurance company practices, treating prostate cancer will continue to involve large sums—and skillful marketers will respond accordingly.

UNDER THE PRIMUS

On day two of my "long march" at the Radiation Oncology Center, I had an actual radiation treatment: the first of forty-two scheduled sessions. I was once again lying on the sheet-covered table when Renato said, "Dr. Massullo is happy with the images we made yesterday, so we're ready to start."

"Okey dokey," I replied dumbly. There was something about lying on one's back under a large machine that was about to dispense 1.8 Grays of photonic energy—the radiation equivalent of almost 1300 chest X-rays—at my pubic region that sucked all the witty rejoinders right out of my brain.

"Now, lie perfectly still," Renato instructed. He provided this instruction at some point during each of my twenty-five sessions under the Primus. Given the photonic energies involved, I was highly motivated to follow his instructions lest I inadvertently cause the wrong cells in my body to be radiated.

There was a period of silence after Renato left the room. I carefully turned my head to stare at the two computer monitors mounted on the wall to my right, making sure everything below my shoulders remained fixed in place. The monitors were too far away for me to see the exact words on the screen, but it was clear that one of them included the same photo that was on my Rad Onc ID card. The remainder of what was on the screen looked like the treatment plan, providing the exact dosage and timing instructions to the Primus. The second screen showed the current shape of the collimator leaves and the angular position of the collimator head.

I heard a muted but highly energetic buzzing sound, not unlike an arc lamp being lit. I knew billions of photons were now flying at me at light speed. Counting "one-one thousand, two-one thousand…" I judged the buzzing to last about eight seconds before it stopped. A few seconds later, the gantry above me containing the collimator head rotated almost noiselessly clockwise ninety degrees and pointed straight at my right hip. There was a brief pause after the gantry halted, and then more buzzing, about the same duration as before. Then silence again, and the head continued its clockwise path. Although I couldn't see it, I could tell from the image on the computer monitor that the collimator head was directly below me, pointing up through the cantilevered table. I now understood why the table was made of a carbon fiber composite material that was invisible to X-rays. This time the buzzing seemed to last a little longer, perhaps ten to twelve seconds, then silence again. After a final ninety-degree rotation, the collimator was now pointed at my left hip. The machine came to life one last time for another eight seconds or so. Now a longer silence followed, but the collimator head remained fixed in this final position. Altogether no more than five minutes had elapsed since Renato had left the room. It all felt distinctly anticlimactic. All these weeks of preparation, implanting, inserting, and testing had culminated in four intervals of a few seconds of subdued buzzing and then silence.

Gretchen appeared around the corner. "Great job, Craig. You did really well." Of course, doing "really well" under the Primus meant doing absolutely nothing at all. "Now that we know everything is lined up and working, let's make those alignment points permanent." She revealed a small pen-like instrument in her right hand and poked it in the center of each of the three black crosses, which she assured me would eventually wear off. With three sharp pinpricks, I had just received my first tattoos at the age of 62. Just three tiny black dots that, like the gold balls in my prostate, I would now carry as permanent souvenirs of my time on the Oncology Adventure Ride.

As the "long march" under the Primus continued, radiotherapy treatments had become my profession. Not only did it consume three hours each weekday, but more importantly, it gave purpose to my days. After all the months of diagnosis and preparation, I was finally doing something about the cancer, even if it was only lying on a rock-hard table for a few minutes. Maybe just showing up day after day was why Gretchen told me, "Great job, Craig." I started to feel the oft-predicted side effects around week three: painful urination, lots of gas, and what might be discreetly termed "bowel irregularity."

Side Effects of Radiotherapy Treatments

The most common side effects of radiation are:

- Skin reaction
- Fatigue

Other, less common side effects are:

- Hair loss
- Nausea and vomiting
- Diarrhea
- Loss of appetite
- Low blood counts

I had changed my diet to avoid grains, salads, and fresh fruit to minimize "roughage" and was consuming what might be called the "white diet." But just as I was adjusting to the radiation routine, it was time to head to a different, somewhat more sophisticated machine: the Novalis.

FOLLOWING THE MONEY

Up to this point in my treatment, it hadn't occurred to me to find out my particular price of admission to the Oncology Adventure Ride. Thus far, I had not been privy to the transactions that had occurred between Pacific Urology and my insurance company. However, John Muir Medical Center had mailed a copy of the bill it had submitted to Blue Cross for radiation performed during the past month. The hospital's invoice worked out to about $3,300 per session under the Primus. While I was pretty sure that Blue Cross would not actually reimburse the hospital's list price, the size of the bill was nonetheless surprising.

Unlike some other cancers, a wide range of prostate cancer treatment options spanning a broad cost spectrum has evolved. Treatments run the gamut from active surveillance (also called "expectant management") to androgen deprivation therapy (ADT) to prostatectomy to radiotherapy, which comes in several varieties. Within the radiation branch there is brachytherapy (placing a number of tiny radioactive "seeds" into the prostate)

How prostate cancer is treated

- Active surveillance (expectant management)
- Radical prostatectomy
  - Open retropubic
  - Laparoscopic
  - Robotic-assisted laparoscopic

- Radiotherapy
  - Electron beam radiotherapy (EBRT)
  - Proton beam radiotherpay (PBRT)
  - Brachytherapy, including high dose rate (HDR) brachytherapy

- Androgen deprivation therapy (ADT). Also called "androgen suppression therapy," or simply, "hormone therapy." ADT is accomplished via pharmaceuticals that are sometimes called testosterone inactivating pharmaceuticals (TIP)
- High frequency ultrasound (HiFU) is practiced in Europe and is currently in clinical trials in the US.

as well as the traditional electron beam radiation therapy that I was undergoing. Radiation may also be used in combination with other treatments, such as radiotherapy along with ADT or brachytherapy together with radiotherapy.

The challenge for both patients and their doctors is that, in terms of their survival rates, treatment options are essentially indistinguishable. A 2009 analysis by the RAND Corporation points out, "No therapy has been shown superior to another." In the view of some dispassionate observers, choosing a prostate cancer treatment is similar to purchasing any other expensive consumer product. Ideally, they suggest, frugal patients with local cancer would opt for active surveillance (expectant management) whenever circumstances warrant. Other patients might choose the popular, middle-of-the road course such as prostatectomy, knowing there are risks of impotence and incontinence. Or, perhaps the doctor and patient might go for the more luxurious alternatives of radiotherapy combined with hormone therapy

(ADT). At the high end of the expense spectrum is proton beam therapy (PBRT), twice as costly as conventional radiotherapy.

One *New York Times* article claimed that,

> *In our current fee-for-service medical system—in which doctors and hospitals are paid for how much care they provide, rather than how well they care for their patients—you can probably guess which treatments are becoming more popular: the ones that cost a lot of money.*

But although cost factors do play a role, they are not the primary determinants of which treatment type the patient ultimately receives. A closer look reveals that it's primarily the age of the patient and the stage of the cancer that determine the selection of treatment method—and therefore, the cost.

Localized prostate cancers, about 80 percent of diagnosed cases, enjoy the greatest range of treatment options, from expectant management, which, not surprisingly, is the least expensive choice, to prostatectomy or radiation. Even ADT, traditionally used only with locally-advanced or metastasized cancers, is now being recommended more frequently for patients with localized cancers, although this practice is controversial since the side effect risks of ADT can easily outweigh the benefits of treating a slow-growing cancer so aggressively. Radiation is usually the preferred treatment course for older men with "co-morbidities" such as diabetes or heart disease where surgery could add excessive stress on the patient and impede his ability to recover. Prostatectomy is more commonly recommended for younger men in their 50s and 60s.

For locally advanced cancers like mine, or where the cancer has metastasized to distant parts of the body, the range of treatment choices narrows. Active surveillance is completely off the table. Surgery would need to extend far beyond the gland itself, thereby reducing the chances of excising all the cancer while simultaneously raising the odds of severe incontinence and impotence. (This was certainly the grim reality in my own case.) Some, although not all, practitioners view brachytherapy as problematic for advanced tumors, because it needs to be combined with other forms of radiation. So, for most men with advanced cancer like mine, the choices pretty much come down to radiotherapy, ADT, or a combination of the two, which is now the recommended treatment for nearly all Stage III and Stage IV cases as it has been proven to be more effective than either method used alone. In general, the therapies for tumors in Stages III and IV are substantially more expensive than those typically used for localized cases.

The costs of treatment options vary. An analysis of long-term costs appeared in a 2007 issue of *Cancer*, titled "Cumulative Cost Comparison of Prostate Cancer Treatments" (hereafter, "CCC"). This paper studied costs in a sample of more than 4,500 newly diagnosed patients across a variety of dimensions, including age, ethnicity, clinical risk for disease progression, and treatment type. The study looked at average costs in 2004 dollars for the first six months of treatment as well as total cost for each treatment type. (The amounts shown in the table are actual "raw costs" and should not be confused with the often inflated amounts that hospitals, doctors, and treatment centers bill insurance companies, who invariably pay much less than the "list price" shown on the bill.)

This study also assessed total cost of each treatment type. ADT turns out to be the most expensive because these are expensive drugs that are administered over several years. Active Surveillance total cost remained the lowest ($32,100) but not by the substantial advantage it had during the first six months, because typically at some point the cancer that is being "actively surveilled" has to be treated.

The CCC authors assess the total societal cost of prostate cancer by asserting that "the impact of treatment on survival is still a matter of much debate, and because of widespread early detection, there has been considerable [upward] stage migration,

Average Treatment Costs

Treatment Type	First 6 Months	Total
Active surveillance:	$2,600	$32,100
Brachytherapy:	$7,600	$35,100
ADT:	$8,800	$69,200
Radiotherapy (EBRT):	$24,200	$59,500
Surgery (RP):	$12,200	$36,900

(PBRT costs were not included in the study)
Note: This analysis was performed in 2009.

resulting in the identification of small-volume, low-grade cancers, many of which may not be associated with progression if left untreated." Translated: PSA screening, digital rectal exams (DREs), and follow-up biopsies allow doctors to detect prostate tumors earlier than ever, but many of them simply don't require immediate treatment, and some may never require treatment. Absent some control mechanism, over-diagnosis leads to over-treatment. Two long-term studies—one in the US and one in Europe—indicated that few lives were saved as a consequence of PSA screening. The sequence from PSA screening to biopsy to treatment with only a small reduction in prostate cancer mortality led the United States Preventive Services Task Force (USPSTF) in 2011 to issue its controversial recommendation to eliminate PSA-based screening for most men. At the individual level, however, thousands of men believe that blood tests indicating a raised PSA value followed by a biopsy led to the detection of cancers that might have killed them without early screening. This controversy will not be resolved until a test that definitively distinguishes between aggressive and indolent cancers becomes available.

Unnecessary expense to society at large is certainly one consequence of over-treatment. Another is the cost to the patient, since incontinence and impotence are a heavy price to pay to remove a tumor that would not ultimately do any serious harm. But for many men, the natural reaction to hearing, "You have prostate cancer" is something like "I don't care about expense or side effects; I just want it out of me. Besides, my insurance covers all the costs." The sentiment about insurance is not a psychological consequence of the diagnosis, but a result of an insurance-based fee-for-treatment system, where the true costs of medical treatment are usually invisible to the patient—at least if he has adequate health insurance. Of course, treatment costs are completely out of reach for the millions of uninsured men in this country, some of whom will be diagnosed (as I was) before the age when Medicare kicks in, another complicated piece of the puzzle.

The 2007 study also estimated the total costs over afive-and-one-half year period for different treatment options. The bottom line of the analysis is that most doctors and patients choose a particular treatment rationally, even though emotion is clearly involved in the decision. The article's authors found that

> *Risk is significantly related to initial treatment choice. Fifty-four percent of all ADTs and 35 percent of all EBRTs [radiotherapy] were given to high-risk men, and they manifested the highest cost treatments over time.*

Contrary to the implication of the *New York Times* article mentioned earlier, which implied that many doctors recommend the treatments that generate the highest revenues, these data suggest that, in general, physicians are assessing a variety of factors, including the patient's age and overall health, the aggressiveness of the tumor, and the risk of recurrence, and prescribing the treatment course likely to be most effective for that particular case.

In all the twists and turns of testing and diagnosis that led to my eventual treatment course, including the unexpected shift from anti-androgen to ADT, I never perceived a revenue maximization agenda on the part of any of the doctors involved. I felt only that they were seeking the most effective treatment for my particular situation. Of course, exceptions to every general rule mean there are doubtless egregious cases where patients have been subjected to treatment courses whose unstated goal was maximizing revenue over medical benefit.

The CCC study also found a correlation between cumulative cost and patient age:

> *Prostate-related cancer treatment costs [across 5.5 years]... are highest for the youngest age group and decrease with increasing age.*

This makes sense, because the younger the patient is, the longer he is likely to be treated—especially if the cancer recurs. In my case, the costs of radiation and ADT constituted my first year of treatment, with ADT-related costs to continue for at least three years, and probably more, depending if and when my cancer becomes castrate resistant and/or eventually metastasizes.

Regardless of how carefully treatments are chosen, treating prostate cancer remains an expensive proposition—at both the individual and collective levels. Over the next twenty years, treating prostate cancer will exact even larger individual and societal costs as the baby boomer generation ages. Over-treatment of this cohort will only add unnecessary cost and suffering. The long-term solution is hardly surprising, as the CCC authors conclude,

> *Obviously, earlier diagnosis of high-risk disease could have a powerful effect on both cost and the more important clinical outcomes (recurrence and survival).*

In other words, if we could reliably distinguish the approximately 15 to 20 percent of high-risk cases like mine that lead to advanced and metastatic cancers, overall cost could be reduced substantially by avoiding unnecessary treatment of slow growing "indolent" cancers. Even better, being able to characterize tumor aggressiveness at the point of diagnosis could not only reduce over-treatment, but would reduce the prostate cancer mortality rate as well. Happily, this is an area that researchers are working on, with much of the focus on identifying genetic markers that may indicate the potential for aggressive cancer more accurately.

However insightful and incisive their analysis, the CCC authors fail to address an increasingly urgent issue: At some point, there may not be enough money to pay for expensive therapies as the population ages. This makes the issue of being able to identify aggressive tumors earlier even more pressing. Cynics may reply that the doctors, medical groups, and companies that profit from prostate cancer treatment will not favor shrinking the potential market. But within discussions about "out of control" costs and demands for reform, it's encouraging to patients that many members of the medical community emphasize that improving survival remains the primary goal. But the cynics are also partially correct. The voices that raise concerns about controlling treatment costs may be just a small oasis of rationality in a desert of increasingly expensive treatment technology.

EIGHT

The Therapeutic Combat Zone

THE DILEMMA OF CHOICE

My friend Don was 68 years old when he was diagnosed with a Gleason 7, T2 tumor in his prostate. Since the cancer appeared to be localized, surgery was an option. Radiotherapy was an equally viable option. Don's urologist, a surgeon, recommended surgery to remove his cancer. Don then visited Dr. Massullo, my radiation oncologist, who described the advantages of radiation, much as he had explained them to me. Don then sought a third opinion from a doctor who specialized in high dose rate (HDR) brachytherapy, which involves temporarily implanting and then removing radioactive needles instead of the permanent implantation of radioactive seeds used in traditional brachytherapy. Not surprisingly, this doctor claimed his approach was superior to other treatments for a person with a localized cancer like Don's.

So, three opinions later, Don was much better informed about his treatment alternatives, but the best path for him was no clearer than before he had met with any of the doctors: Each had recommended his particular specialty. Like so many other men, Don was left to sort out by himself which treatment would be best for him. Knowing he already had a heart condition, he was unwilling to risk surgery. The HDR brachytherapy seemed too new and untested for his comfort level, so he opted for radiotherapy.

Don's experience is typical. Each doctor understands his or her treatment specialty better than the alternatives, and therefore is most comfortable recommending it. In addition, Don's treatment choice was also indirectly affected by the behind-the-scenes competition among equipment manufacturers, pharmaceutical companies, service providers, and consultants seeking to maximize profits.

The battles over treatment alternatives are being fought mainly out of the patient's view in professional journals and conference presentations. Dr. Deborah A. Kuban, Professor at the MD Anderson Cancer Center, criticizes this state of affairs, stating,

> *So here we go again with one more round in the battle of treatment options for localized prostate cancer. While more than three decades of such sparring has gotten us no closer to evidence-based conclusions, one might say that these matches do serve the purpose of bringing out the best and the worst of the therapeutic contenders.*

Kuban also remarks that numerous studies have repeatedly demonstrated that no single treatment is clearly superior to the others. She argues,

> *It's time to work in a multidisciplinary manner to help patients make treatment decisions based on their particular set of tumor, medical, psychological, and social circumstances, while using clinical studies to collect comparative information and quality-of-life data.*

In Kuban's ideal world, Don would have been served in a single, multi-disciplinary setting including an urologist, radiation oncologist, and medical oncologist. This group could have assisted Don in weighing the pros and cons of each treatment option based on the particulars of his case. Don would not have had to make three separate office visits to hear three independent medical opinions. Most importantly, he would not have been left completely on his own to make his treatment decision. Multidisciplinary settings like these exist at a few cancer centers, but in general, patients must seek information and make treatment decisions on their own.

Kuban hopes

> *...that we continue to have the luxury to do this [multidisciplinary approach], and that future treatment decisions are not based more on cost than on the patients' best interests.*

However, given the conflicts within each of the three treatment arenas themselves, as well as looming healthcare policy issues, it's difficult to be optimistic.

SCALPELS AT 20 PACES

While surgery permanently separates a man from his cancerous prostate, the procedure is hardly risk-free. Before 1982, when Dr. Patrick Walsh developed the nerve-sparing technique, men who underwent a radical prostatectomy were almost always left with permanent impotence and often incontinence as well. Before then, radiation was the preferred treatment, since it produced fewer permanent side effects. But after Walsh demonstrated that a prostate could be removed while sparing delicate nerves and avoiding the dreaded "I" words, surgery became more popular, eventually replacing radiotherapy as the "gold standard" treatment for localized prostate cancer.

Since 75 to 80 percent of prostate cancer cases are localized, it's not unreasonable for a recent editorial to claim,

> *We believe that for the majority of patients with organ-confined prostate cancer, radical prostatectomy (RP) remains the gold standard with respect to both oncologic success and maximization of quality of life.*

The authors of this article go on to list the advantages of radical prostatectomy over radiotherapy and brachytherapy, including better urinary, bowel, and sexual function, concluding that,

RP has stood the test of time for the treatment of prostate cancer, which is reflected in current choices for prostate cancer intervention: 51% of patients undergo RP, 6% EBRT, and 13% observation. ... RP is likely to remain the gold standard for the foreseeable future.

Although this group of physicians may agree that surgery is the way to go, conflict arises within the surgical community over the method by which RP should be performed. One group of surgeons—let's call them "Walsh traditionalists"—perform classical open surgery, manually using their scalpels to conduct "radical retropubic prostatectomy" (RRP), also known as "open" RP. Since the 1990s, however, open RP has largely given way to minimally invasive laparoscopic surgery, which involves a smaller incision and the use of fiber optics to provide a visual field to the surgeon without opening up the abdomen. Its advantages over open RP are less bleeding, a shorter hospital stay, and faster recovery.

Taking laparoscopic surgery to its next logical step are the "Silicon Valley technologists" who perform "robot assisted laparoscopic prostatectomy" (RALP), using the daVinci Surgical System developed by Intuitive Surgical, Inc. Introduced in the early 2000s, RALP is lauded by its proponents to be the most sophisticated surgical option available. About 17,500 men received RALP in 2005, a number that rose to more than 60,000 per year in 2008 and 2009—which is more than 30% of the total prostate cancer diagnoses for those years. Long-term outcomes are the important point of comparison, though, and RALP has not been around long enough to demonstrate superior outcomes at ten years out and therefore cannot claim to be the "gold standard" of surgery just yet.

Nevertheless, RALP promoters claim that current results

... suggest a rapid recovery with the robotic approach, and a more rapid return of continence has been our observation as well. Similarly, 12-month potency data are also favorable (70% to 80%) with the robotic approach and comparable to even longer term (24 months) data of expert open [surgery] series (47% to 76%).

These surgeons believe that RALP will soon replace traditional open surgery, claiming,

> *A rapidly growing body of evidence is showing that the
> robotic approach measures up to the past and present stan-
> dards for radical prostatectomy and, with certain benefits
> of decreased blood loss and lower morbidity, the robotic
> approach may soon represent a new surgical standard of care
> for the treatment of localized prostate cancer.*

The technologists have put the traditionalists on the defen-
sive, who in turn are questioning these calls for a speedy transition
to robotics. Implying that excellent marketing and shiny new
technology are seducing men to select RALP, the traditionalists
argue,

> *Nowhere on the website [touting RALP] was surgeon or
> site-specific outcome data provided to support the aforemen-
> tioned marketing statements.*

These traditionalists claim that either technique (RRP or RALP)
has comparable outcomes:

> *There were no significant differences in early or late complica-
> tions, 1-year continence rates, potency and positive surgical
> margin rate. Most importantly the 3-year progression-free
> survival rate was equivalent (92.4% for RRP vs. 92.2% for
> RALP).*

Thus, the traditionalists conclude,

> *[Robotic surgery] has not yet become the firmly established
> standard of care because long-term outcomes have yet to be
> established.*

From the patient's point of view, the only useful information
to emerge from these statistics is that, as usual, no single treatment approach, including the two popular forms of RP surgery,

has been demonstrated to be definitively superior to any other. So, while the surgeons continue to argue about details behind the scenes, a patient's most rational decision may be less difficult than it first appears. If open surgery and robotic-assisted surgery have essentially the same outcomes in terms of success, then it's probably best to follow the advice of my friend John, who underwent prostate surgery a few years ago: "A successful outcome of this operation depends 90 to 99 percent on the skill of the surgeon. Find a surgeon who's done this operation before—a lot."

As with any other custom-built product, it is not whether the builder uses hand tools or power tools. What really counts are the skills and experience of the craftsman.

PHARMA CORNUCOPIA

While competing surgical options dominate the treatment of most localized Stage II prostate cancers, the therapeutic drug and radiation industries dominate the treatment of Stage III and IV cancers. Thousands of men with advanced prostate cancer (including me) would benefit from advances in therapeutic drugs, both in terms of decreased side effects and increased longevity. The major question is: Can pharmaceutical progress be delivered at a reasonable cost?

One area ripe for innovation is hormone therapy, which employs drugs that are rather awkwardly termed "testosterone inactivating pharmaceuticals" (TIP). Androgen deprivation therapy (ADT) reduces testosterone to "castrate levels," effectively halting cancer growth—at least for a while. However, the absence of testosterone in a man's body creates numerous adverse effects, "including obesity, insulin resistance and lipid alterations as well as the association … with diabetes and cardiovascular disease." These effects can be so significant that some researchers have seriously questioned the risk-benefit tradeoffs of using ADT at all, and especially as a treatment for localized prostate cancers. Other researchers have advocated the use of anti-androgens such as bicalutamide (Casodex®) in lieu of ADT. This approach is called "anti-androgen monotherapy" (AAM) because anti-androgens allow testosterone to remain in the blood stream, thereby avoiding the effects associated with its suppression. However, early research indicates that the survival rates of men on AAM may not be as favorable as those on traditional ADT.

Side effects aside, the major shortcoming of ADT using TIP is that it inevitably loses its ability to halt the cancer's progression. The length of time ADT will effectively suppress cancer in an individual man is impossible to predict. It may be as short as two years, or it may be a decade or more before the patient develops castrate-resistant prostate cancer (CRPC). At this point, so-called "second line" treatments are usually prescribed. Often, an antifungal drug called ketoconazole, usually administered together with hydrocortisone, can be useful in lowering testosterone levels after ADT has failed. A drug approved by the FDA in 2011, Zytiga® (abiraterone), operates by inhibiting an enzyme involved in testosterone production and appears to have fewer severe side effects than ketoconozole. Other drugs such as MDV3100 (still in the FDA approval pipeline as of this writing) promise even more effective inhibition of the androgen receptor in cancerous prostate cells than existing anti-androgen drugs. At this point, Zytiga is approved only for use after chemotherapy, although many doctors are prescribing it "off label" for use before chemo.

Regardless of when they're used, the cost of these new pharmaceuticals is substantial. The list price of Zytiga is approximately $5,000 per month, while the older drug ketoconozole costs just a few dollars each month. There is little reason to expect that newer, even more effective drugs such as MDV3100 will be less expensive than Zytiga.

Once a man becomes castrate resistant, his prostate cancer almost always advances to Stage IV, and the cancer tends to metastasize painfully in the bones, although it can metastasize to other organs such as the kidneys and liver as well. It is at this point that traditional chemotherapy usually comes into play. The usual first choice for prostate cancer chemotherapy is Taxotere® (docetaxel). Like all chemotherapy agents, it will slow, but not halt, the progression of the disease, on average extending survival by several months. In 2010, a new chemotherapy agent, Jevtana® (cabazitaxel), joined the group of chemotherapy drugs approved for prostate cancer. However, each man's prostate cancer is unique. Different men respond differently to different combinations of hormone and chemotherapy agents. And all these chemo drugs invariably require additional drugs such as prednisone to control the substantial side effects of the treatment. Finding the appropriate "mix" requires an oncologist experienced in treating advanced prostate cancer. Several cancer research groups are developing genetic profiling techniques that will assist oncologists in coming up with the best combination and sequence of treatment agents for individual cases.

Chemotherapy may be effective, but it is hard on the body, since it injures healthy cells along with the cancer cells it is designed to annihilate. Looking to harness the body's own immune system to help fight off the cancer, a completely new approach called autologous cellular immunotherapy has been developed to treat men with late stage cancers. With immunotherapy, the patient contributes his own blood, which is sent to the pharmaceutical factory, where it is combined with the drug, which in effect "trains" the patient's own immune system T-cells to recognize and fight cancer cells. The drug is then infused back into the patient, where the newly empowered T-cells go to work. Provenge® (sipuleucel-T) was developed for patients with metastatic CRPC, and it is the first FDA-approved immunotherapy drug for any cancer. Other drugs with these vaccine-like qualities are in the development and testing stages.

As with Zytiga and other androgen receptor inhibitor drugs, the economic downside of Provenge is that a single therapeutic course costs almost $100,000. From a coldly analytical point of view, the drug may or may not be a wise investment. The FDA trial results showed that Provenge resulted in an average four-month extension of life for patients with Stage IV prostate cancer. The question becomes: As increasing numbers of men seek this therapy—and other expensive pharmaceuticals such as Zytiga and MDV3100—who pays and how much? Since the majority of men with prostate cancer are older than 65, Medicare payment policies will play an enormous role in determining the future of cutting-edge therapeutics such as Provenge.

Eager to sell their wares to drug researchers and potential investors, market research organizations forecast ever-increasing profitability for this growing prostate cancer treatment market. A press release for a new study from Decision Resources, Inc. puts it bluntly,

Prostate cancer a booming market for new therapies, [with] a sustained annual growth of more than 3.4% in sales of prostate cancer therapies [drugs] from 2005 to 2015 will be driven primarily by new entries to the market that will add to, rather than replace existing therapies…Novel agents with proven benefits have huge potential and could add an impressive $1.5 billion in annual sales to this underserved market.

Drug Pipeline Update remarks on this growth from another angle,

There are today no less than 300 therapeutics targeting prostate cancer in active development, from early preclinical to marketed drugs.

Whether or not it is an unconscious admission of the potential problem all this market growth may create, one press release concludes with a surprisingly candid admission,

In a market already flooded with pharmaceuticals, the number of alternatives is only projected to increase—not necessarily an ideal situation for doctors already hard-pressed to stay abreast of which drugs to recommend to patients.

Out of all this research, investment, and marketing rhetoric, new drug-based therapies will continue to emerge. However, given that clinical trials needed for FDA approval can take several years, some of these drugs will benefit only those men yet to be diagnosed several years hence. But one wonders if simply "add[ing] to, rather than replac[ing] existing therapies" is a beneficial strategy for doctors prescribing these drugs and the men receiving them. Will these doctors and patients be viewed by the pharmaceutical industry simply as faceless revenue sources that will be forced to choose among a growing array of therapeutic alternatives whose comparative long-term advantages are still unknown? Or will pharmaceutical companies view patients as individual men, some of whom face difficult choices between expensive treatment or an earlier death?

We can also ask if there is a risk of ending up with too many pharmaceutical alternatives in the name of market competition and profit. Many men with prostate cancer are already confused by the array of drugs available for the treatment of advanced disease, and the sequence in which they ideally should be used. Even worse, many of their oncologists are also confused. Advanced prostate cancer is a frustratingly complex disease, and every patient's case is unique. For some, Zytiga is virtually a wonder drug. For other men, it has no effect. This is true for virtually every pharmaceutical therapy. What efforts will the profit-driven pharmaceutical industry make to communicate the complex realities of each of their drugs?

Or will health insurance and government policies decide that the cost-benefit ratios of new pharmaceuticals are simply too unattractive to merit payment (usually via Medicare) as increasing numbers of baby boomers are diagnosed? In the absence of reimbursement for expensive therapeutic treatments, the problem would then becomes not too many choices, but too few, as dwindling investments in research and development lead to fewer new therapies to choose from. For men with advanced prostate cancer, all these possibilities loom darkly on the horizon.

RADIATION WARS

The surgical and therapeutic drug markets appear relatively peaceful compared to the conflict raging among alternative radiation treatment technologies. Market positions are rapidly being claimed, and enormous sums of money are at stake. Advocates for improving traditional electron beam radiotherapy (EBRT), an X-ray technology that has been in use since the early twentieth century, stand on the one side of the battlefield, and proton beam radiotherapy (PBRT) proponents occupy the opposing camp. This profit-driven battle too often obscures the men (and women) with cancer needing treatment.

There is even conflict within the EBRT community itself. Intensity-modulated radiotherapy (IMRT) and its newer variants, image-guided radiotherapy (IGRT) and tomotherapy, are recent EBRT developments. IMRT has come into wide use during the last ten years. IGRT is a subset of IMRT and takes real-time X-ray images of gold seeds inserted in the prostate, using software to adjust beam placement even more precisely than traditional IMRT systems. Tomotherapy delivers radiation "slice by slice," claiming greater accuracy in its delivery. All these methods use sophisticated computer algorithms to control beam intensity and to focus the high-energy photons more accurately on the cancer site, while avoiding nearby healthy tissue. The prostate's location deep inside the pelvis makes this a challenging task. IMRT and its siblings (hereafter lumped in the IMRT category) have substantially reduced—but not completely eliminated—the bowel and urinary side effects associated with earlier forms of EBRT.

IMRT has proven useful beyond treating prostate cancer; IGRT is especially effective for treating inoperable brain tumors. But these newer technologies are expensive. Depending on accessories, a typical IMRT system costs between $1 million and $2 million. An IGRT system is about $4 million. Tomotherapy is in a similar cost ballpark. They all have high operating costs as well, since in addition to the radiation oncologist, radiotherapy also requires an experienced physicist to develop and program the patient's treatment plan, as well as skilled technicians to operate the machines and administer the actual therapy. Add up these costs and radiation therapy of any kind becomes an expensive proposition.

Advocates of IMRT have been quick to respond to criticisms about its relative cost effectiveness:

> *Although more expensive [than older 3D conformal radiation therapy], our study found IMRT to be cost-effective for men with intermediate-risk prostate cancer because it improved the quality-adjusted survival [rate]...*

was the conclusion of a presentation made at a 2004 meeting of the American Society of Therapeutic Radiology and Oncology (ASTRO). Later, the same presenter claimed,

> *Higher doses of radiation could be given with potentially greater quality-adjusted survival because of fewer side effects from IMRT.*

The same cost-benefit arguments will undoubtedly also be applied to more costly technologies such as IGRT and tomotherapy as they come into wider use.

However, some critics assert that urologists have a conflict of interest when they prescribe IMRT in lieu of less expensive treatment options because their practices stand to profit from that choice. In 2006, *The New York Times* reported that a number of urological practices bought IMRT equipment and then proceeded to prescribe radiation therapy to their patients, thereby profiting handsomely. According to the article, one IMRT packager promises:

> *Join the Urorad team and let us show your group how Urorad clients double their practice's revenue.*

A critic quoted in the *Times* article noted, "It's not illegal to do this, [but] that doesn't make it right." If patients are aware of this, they are forced to add another layer of concern to their already worrisome situation: Does the urologist have the patient's best interests at heart, or are there additional unspoken financial motives at work? It's not unreasonable to conclude that in some (hopefully small) percentage of cases, financial issues might influence the doctor's recommended treatment.

The controversies surrounding cost justification and profits from IMRT, IGRT, and other new technologies pale in comparison to the real battle: traditional EBRT versus proton beam radio therapy (PBRT). Conceptually, both technologies do the same thing: direct high energies at cancer cells such that they die when the cells try to reproduce. EBRT uses photons while proton beam radiotherapy (PBRT) uses protons. The technical advantage of PBRT over EBRT is that the heavier mass of protons allows for more precise placement of energy directly into the cancerous cells, minimizing damage to healthy surrounding tissue. PBRT has proven most effective for some rare spine, brain, and eye tumors, as well as for children, whose healthy tissues are much more sensitive to damage caused by radiation. And, as Dr. Massullo had pointed out when I asked, PBRT is well suited for oddly shaped tumors, such as those surrounding the eye socket.

A PBRT installation costs a staggering $150 million. In 2010, there were eight active PBRT centers in the US, with two more under construction, and others in the planning stages. Investors are attracted to PBRT because a center running 16 hours a day, 6 days a week, can generate $50 million in annual revenue, with $18 million in pretax profits. And it is prostate cancer that generates the serious cash. PBRT advocates predict that because there are fewer side effects, and because of the precise nature of proton beam radiation, even higher doses of radiation could extend the survival rates for patients with advanced prostate cancer.

Critics of PBRT claim these advantages are only theoretical, arguing,

> *There have been no randomized trials directly comparing the efficacy and tolerability of high-dose PBRT with equally high-dose IMRT in the treatment of clinically localized-prostate cancer.*

Given the absence of data, most researchers hypothesize that the long-term outcomes of protons and photons are similar, except that PBRT costs twice as much as conventional radiotherapy. One study concluded,

> *PBRT was not cost effective for most patients with prostate cancer when using the commonly accepted benchmark of $50,000 quality-adjusted life years.*

Another study noted,

> *Only a small population of men with intermediate-risk prostate cancer will benefit [from PBRT] in terms of cost effectiveness using the current definition of cost effectiveness.*

Nevertheless, men with generous health insurance benefits, as well as wealthy foreigners, continue to flock to PBRT centers for a typical eight- to nine-week course. In my own situation, PBRT was not a sensible option for several reasons. But if it had been (and if my insurance company had agreed to cover the cost), I wonder if I could have done the same sort of dispassionate economic analysis advocated by the study's authors? And would I have decided to forego PBRT simply because I had concluded it was not cost effective? Separating one's emotional desire to receive what some believe to be the most effective treatment with the least side effects from economic reality is a thorny task.

This conflict of emotion and rationality was amply reflected in the 2009 controversy over whether women should start to get mammograms at age 40 or 50. Emotion says that, if starting to test at 40 instead of 50 saves just one life, it is worth the cost. But economics and statistics say that the benefit of that one life saved is not worth the total expense of testing thousands of perfectly healthy younger women, concluding that 50 is the preferred age at which to start testing.

In the case of prostate cancer, the 2011 recommendation by the United States Preventive Services Task Force that PSA tests not be routinely used as a screening tool creates a similar dilemma. At the coldly statistical level at which public health recommendations are decided, the proposal to eliminate universal screening may be rational and logical. But thousands of men believe—the majority of them correctly—that their lives were saved when PSA screening led to further tests that detected cancer, which could then be treated. As far as they are concerned, the alternative to PSA screening would have been an earlier, painful death.

As of 2010, no large-scale trial comparing the long-term effectiveness of PBRT versus EBRT had yet been conducted, although several were in the offing. At this writing, any claim of superiority by either camp has been based on little more than subjective assertion. The disagreement over which treatment should prevail, together with the massive sums of money involved in constructing and operating a proton beam therapy center led Anthony Zeitman at the Massachusetts General Hospital (which already has a PBRT installation) to predict some form of imminent economic disaster. Writing in the *Journal of Clinical Oncology*, with an editorial titled "The Titanic and the Iceberg: Prostate Proton Therapy and Health Care Economics," he argues that

> *The expansive vigor of medical innovation is heading inexorably toward the harsh reality of economic fact. The controversial treatment of prostate cancer epitomizes this clash. ... Sailing forward, powered by the winds of advocacy, of market forces, and of high-stakes investment, is proton*

[beam] therapy, the proud vanguard of modern technology. Elsewhere, waiting patiently in the darkness, are the hard, cold, unyielding laws of economics.

While PBRT may be at the technological vanguard, the warning is equally applicable, if somewhat further out in time, to therapeutic drugs, conventional radiotherapy, robotic surgery, and an emerging assortment of newer prostate cancer treatments, such as cryoablation and ultrasonics.

A growing market and untrammeled competition will doubtless yield innovative therapies, but there are always consequences. As Dr. Zeitman warns,

If there is no advantage, unless the costs change dramatically, proton therapy cannot be judged worth the price for localized prostate cancer.

Since prostate cancer occurs most often in older men, Medicare reimbursements have historically made up a large proportion of total payments for treatment. It would take only a relatively modest change in reimbursement policies to drastically alter the economic picture. Investors in PBRT centers could easily find themselves echoing the experience of highly leveraged homeowners, circa 2008.

Drug research funding could dry up as pharmaceutical companies fail to see sufficient profits for their expensive research and development projects. Likewise, hospitals may not see the economic advantage of investing in expensive robotically-assisted surgical equipment. Zeitman concludes his editorial with a grim warning,

Now is not the time to be rearranging the deck chairs but a time to consider redirecting the ship. If we fail to give this issue our attention, then we may have a 21st-century collision between technology and the iceberg, with the same sorry end.

However, there is no law that says improvements in prostate cancer treatment can occur only at ever-increasing cost. There are numerous industries, most notably in semiconductors and computing, where technology has provided ever-increasing performance with ever-decreasing cost. As noted earlier, one enormous cost containment advance in prostate cancer diagnosis and treatment would be the ability to distinguish between aggressive and slow-growing tumors. Perhaps the time has come to focus on these less expensive research developments, before patients find themselves the unwilling victims of an economic crash brought on by overinvestment in expensive technologies.

UNDER THE NOVALIS

"Well, Craig, I'll miss seeing you every day," Renato remarked as he came around the corner into the treatment room just as the Primus had completed its orbit around my pelvis. I had completed twenty-five sessions in twenty-seven days, counting the two days I showed up when the Primus was off-line for repairs. The time seemed to have passed at once in an eternity and an instant. An eternity, because by the sixth week of treatment, I felt like I had been commuting to the Radiation Oncology Center most of my life. An instant, because in trusting my life to the experienced skill of the medical staff, I had formed an intimate relationship with them. It was not a bond of friendship. It was certainly not a bond of shared experience. Only another person who has lain perfectly still under a large machine as it circumnavigates his body dispensing megavolt photons to his nether regions can really know those feelings. Rather, it was more like the bond that evolves when two strangers sit down in the same train compartment and accompany each other on a long journey, passing the time with pleasant conversation. Renato had been my companion in the Primus treatment room for almost six weeks, showing me the ropes of exactly how to crawl onto the treatment table, how to lie perfectly still, how to hold the blue plastic "donut" over my chest that kept my arms positioned up out of the way, and how to make sure the table had been fully lowered before trying to climb off. More importantly, his wry humor had relaxed me, and helped me to endure the entire process with some sense of dignity. I would miss Renato.

The IMRT Primus treatments were analogous to a wide-angle camera lens: They covered a relatively large territory of my pelvis. As Dr. Massullo had explained earlier, this would make sure the area outside my prostate that may have harbored free-floating cancer cells, including the urethra, sphincter and nearby lymph nodes, were sufficiently treated. Now, for the final seventeen sessions, I would be receiving high-energy radiation aimed straight at my prostate gland—a much smaller target using image-guided technology. For that process, I would be treated on the Novalis, the radiotherapy equivalent of a telephoto lens.

The next day Gretchen appeared at the door of the patient's waiting area, smiled, and said, "Hi, Craig, it's a new table for one." I followed her into the Novalis treatment room. This room was smaller than the one that housed the Primus. Varian Medical System's Novalis Tx™, its official moniker, decked out in bright yellow trim, looked to be of a more recent vintage, and less imposingly Germanic than the Primus. It had the same basic architecture as the Siemens machine: a collimator head mounted on a rotating gantry. The intriguing word "BrainLab" was inscribed on the back of the machine. The treatment table looked identical to the one under the Primus, although as I was to find out shortly, it had a few surprises of its own. As I clambered up onto the table, I noticed an array of video cameras mounted on the wall opposite the machine. In the Primus room there had been a single camera to monitor the patient, and I assumed one of the cameras here had the same function. As for the other cameras, their purpose remained a mystery for now. As in the Primus treatment room, there were two computer monitors mounted on the far wall, and two others sitting on a bench immediately to my right of the treatment table. Mounted on posts attached to the ceiling—one to the right of the table, the other on the left—were two metal rectangles about the size of a standard flat screen computer monitor, but without the display. Based on my Internet research, I knew these were the X-ray sensors that the Novalis used to carry out its "image guided" capabilities. Each sensor plate was angled slightly, and when I entered the room I had seen two holes in the floor—again on both sides of the table—slightly behind the machine. These were the X-ray sources that communicated to the sensors jutting down from the ceiling. The emitter in the floor on my right was angled up to the ceiling-mounted sensor on my left, and the floor-mounted source on my left was aimed up at the sensor on the right. The table—and my body—lay directly in the path of both X-ray sources and their corresponding sensors.

Shari joined Gretchen in the treatment room and handed me the familiar blue "donut" to hold with both hands, keeping my arms out of the way of the X-rays. Gretchen also placed a small cloverleaf-shaped aluminum plate attached to a short rod into a metal socket down at the end of the table.

After adjusting the metal cloverleaf, she slid the table—and me—closer to the back of the machine so the collimator head was in its familiar position directly above my pelvis. I saw the usual red laser lines intersecting my body at right angles. "I need a tug," Gretchen said, as Shari pulled on the sheet slightly. Each tech had a black Sharpie marker and they inscribed new black crosses, one on each hip. That evening when I examined them I saw they were about two inches below the tattoo marks inscribed for the Primus. The following day, those black crosses became my fourth and fifth tattoo marks.

"Okay," Gretchen said, "This first session will take a little longer than usual since we need to make sure the robotics are aligned." I wasn't quite sure what this meant, but I knew it had to do with making sure all those high energy photons were aimed squarely at my prostate—and nowhere else.

I lay there perfectly still as I had been instructed. Suddenly, the table moved, tilting my body longitudinally so that my head was now a few inches lower than my feet. Simultaneously, it canted a bit to the left so that my right shoulder was raised slightly higher than my left. During my research about how the Novalis worked, I had assumed the collimator head would be adjusted to me, not the other way around. However, since I was much smaller and lighter than the collimator mounted on its heavy gantry, it didn't take much thought to understand the engineering logic of a robotically controlled six-axis treatment table.

"We should have warned you the table was going to move." Shari had materialized at the foot of the table. "So that's what the aluminum cloverleaf is for," I replied. "It's a target you guys use to adjust me to the machine." I now understood the purpose of the other cameras mounted on the wall: They used the cloverleaf as a reference point, measured the relative position of the table to the machine and adjusted it accordingly.

"Right. Now we're going to X-ray your prostate and make sure we can image the famous gold seeds," Shari said as she left the room. Ah, the gold seeds: After so many weeks, I had almost forgotten they were still there. Now, at long last, they were about to serve their intended purpose as navigational markers for the IGRT system. I heard a solenoid click, followed by the usual X-ray buzzing. It was one of the positioning X-ray sources being activated. I turned my head to the right to get a better view of the computer monitors. X-ray images of an indistinct gray mass, apparently my prostate, materialized on the screen. More fascinating were three small white circles, forming the vertices of a virtual triangle right in the middle of the image. I remembered that X-ray images are seen in the negative and that the white circles were actually a solid mass impervious to X-rays. There was no question that these were the gold seeds. Another solenoid clicked and more buzzing. Now a second, similar image appeared next to the first with the same three white balls, but each in a slightly different position. Two images on the screen: one taken from right to left; the other from left to right. I knew enough about spatial geometry that three points define a plane, and that with the two images, each taken from a different angle, the exact geographic location of the three balls—and therefore of my prostate—could be located in three-dimensional space relative to the location of the machine's collimator head. I presumed this location calculation task was a function of the BrainLab software.

I saw a cursor move onto each of the three points in each image as the software drew lines between the points to form a visual triangle on the monitor. Calculations complete, the table shifted slightly as the computer-driven robotics adjusted the last few millimeters into the exact position. I was now aligned to the machine that stood ready to aim its photons precisely at a tiny organ located deep inside me. The collimator head came to life and began rotating clockwise around my pelvis. If we designated the position of the collimator directly overhead as "north," it had now rotated all the way down to the southeast compass point, pointing back up at me from beneath my right side. A relay clicked, and the familiar buzzing commenced. Its duration was much longer than the Primus, lasting about 90 seconds. The buzzing stopped, and a few seconds later the head moved counterclockwise to due east and stopped. The click-buzz-silence sequence repeated itself through seven points of the compass: east, northeast, north, northwest, west as the collimator traced its arc, ending at the southwest. Only due south—directly underneath the table—was omitted.

The entire process took about eighteen minutes. Shari reappeared in the treatment room. "Good job." The radiation techs were always encouraging when I managed to lay perfectly still, something I was pretty skilled at by this point in the radiotherapy process. After she removed the cloverleaf target and lowered the table, I hopped off.

"See you tomorrow, guys," I said as I headed back to the patient's changing area.

NINE

But Where Are All the Light Blue Ribbons?

RADIATION END GAME

Twenty-six, twenty-seven, twenty-eight completed. Sixteen, fifteen, fourteen to go. Another man that I met in the patient's waiting area had advised me not to count how many sessions were complete—or how many I still had to go. But I could not resist counting both forward and backward each day that I sat in the cramped room waiting for Renato, Gretchen, or Shari to invite me back to the table for one.

Almost everyone who sat in the radiation waiting room looked to be dancing with cancer. I saw only a few, who by their resigned faces, seemed to have become cancer victims. Some patients were young; most were older like me. The women usually wore gowns instead of their blouses, while still wearing their street attire from the waist down. The gown was usually the sign of breast cancer. Men like me, wearing pajama bottoms, were the prostate cancer patients. Men in gowns were there for various upper body cancers: neck and lung mostly. Some of the other patients I met in the waiting room had just completed a course of chemo and were now undergoing radiotherapy. Even worse, others were experiencing chemo and radiation simultaneously. These were the people that helped me realize that I had gotten off pretty easily, all things considered. One lady showed me where the radiation had burned the skin around her shoulders. One older gentleman told me he had radiation for prostate cancer twenty years previously, and was now back because the cancer had reappeared, this time in his pelvic bone. "Hey," he said, "I had twenty great years. I watched my grandchildren grow up. I'm grateful for the time the radiation gave me."

As radiotherapy continues, insurance regulations insist on a weekly meeting with the radiation oncologist. Susan and I met with Dr. Massullo every Wednesday afternoon for ten to fifteen minutes. As the cumulative radiation mounted, the reason for these meetings that had seemed superfluous at first now became apparent. Starting around session fourteen or fifteen, I began to experience some significant side effects. For me, the most severe was a stinging, decreased flow while urinating. It felt like my urethra was swelling and closing up a little more after each day's session.

Thirty-five, thirty-six, thirty-seven completed. By this time, urination was quite painful, so Dr. Massullo prescribed a classic nostrum for the problem, phenazopyridine, a drug that's been around since the early twentieth century. I marveled at its notable side effect as I watched my urine turn fluorescent orange. But it didn't do much to reduce the pain.

Thirty-eight, thirty-nine, forty completed. With just two more sessions in the radiation course left, Susan and I had our last Wednesday meeting with Dr. Massullo. I voiced my concern about how increasingly difficult urination had become.

"Oh, I think everything will be fine," he replied. "Only about three percent of cases actually get a stricture where the urethra closes up altogether—and that usually happens about two to three months after radiation has ended."

Forty-one complete, just one more to go. Driving home that afternoon, I was in a cheery mood. The lengthy daily commute was finally coming to an end. "Just one more session. No sweat," I thought.

Fatigue is a major side effect of radiotherapy, and I headed to bed around nine o'clock that evening. Waking up a little before eleven with the predictable urge to pee, I crawled out of bed and headed to the bathroom. But no matter how hard I tried, nothing would come out. Sitting or standing made no difference. Waiting for another five minutes and trying again didn't help. Another five minutes and still the same: no go.

"Susan, I need to get to the emergency room," I whispered, urgently poking my sleeping wife.

"Huh? What?"

"I can't pee. It's completely closed up."

"Oh," she mumbled, as she returned to consciousness. We both hastily threw on our clothes and stumbled out to the garage. "You need to drive," I announced through the haze of my increasingly desperate urgency.

Drive she did, racing down deserted streets and on to the freeway. It was at once the shortest and longest drive ever made from our house to the hospital twenty-five miles away. Shortest, since Susan made a typically forty minute drive in under thirty-two minutes. Still, from my perspective, it was the longest ride, because my only thought was, "My God, I need relief. When will we ever get there?"

The clerk at the emergency room admitting desk assessed my situation matter-of-factly as I stood squirming anxiously at the check-in desk. The bureaucratic formalities required of someone who walks into an ER rather than arriving by ambulance seemed to take forever.

"What is your address? May I see your insurance card? Do you have a signed healthcare directive?" Given my situation, her questions felt more like a cruel stalling tactic than an administrative necessity.

I glanced around and saw that things were pretty quiet in the ER, so I could hope that once I was admitted, help would be shortly at hand. Susan, who had gone to park the car, appeared at the desk and confirmed the urgency of our mission. I don't remember the clerk's reply, since my attention was focused exclusively on my bladder.

At last (it was probably no more than a minute, but distress had slowed my mental clock almost to a standstill), the triage nurse led me to an exam room. I undressed hastily, put on the requisite gown, and climbed onto the gurney. She took my pulse (over 100) and blood pressure (195 over 131—an all time record).

She carefully typed all these data into the computer beside the gurney. She began asking what medications I was taking. I knew those records were already on a computer down in the Radiation Oncology Center and told her so. "Sorry, we can't access those records," she replied. I fumed inwardly as I verbally repeated the litany of pharmaceutical names and dosages. Intellectually, I knew this information was necessary, but in addition to the agony spreading throughout my pelvic region, I now had a splitting headache. How much longer would this interrogation continue before both ends of me exploded? Susan, intuitively understanding my anxiety, took my hand and squeezed it. "Just a few more minutes," she said reassuringly. Her loving touch was immensely comforting as the triage nurse departed, saying, "The ER nurse will be right with you."

The registered nurse, whose name badge read "Scott," appeared at the door a minute or two later. "Hi, sounds like you're in some distress," he said brightly as he walked over to the computer and began typing. I began reciting my history without prompting. "I have advanced prostate cancer, and have completed forty-one sessions of radiation down at Rad Onc," I reported, as he continued to type. "I told Doctor Massullo yesterday that it was getting increasingly difficult to pee. 'Difficult' has now become 'impossible.'" Without a word, Scott kept on typing.

"I'll be gone just a minute to get you a Foley catheter," he said, as he turned away from the computer and headed out the door.

He reappeared after a few more agonizing minutes, holding a package wrapped in white paper. He removed the wrapping, carefully separating the various pieces with agonizing slowness. Finally, after applying disinfectant, he inserted it. There was an odd combination of discomfort and urgency. But as he began to inflate the balloon that holds the catheter in place, intense pain overwhelmed everything else. Scott could tell by looking at my face that this was not going well. "I can't get the balloon to inflate," he said as he pulled out the rubber tube. "I think we need to try a smaller cath," he said as he left the room.

He returned a few minutes later holding another white package and performed the same unwrapping and disinfection ceremony. Time stood still. "It's in," he said at last. The plastic bag at the other end of the catheter filled and relief engulfed me.

"It worked!" Susan exclaimed. She didn't need to say another thing. I loved her—and Dr. Foley's invention, as well.

As my bladder emptied and my head cleared, I glanced at the clock. It was almost one in the morning, a little more than two hours since I had awakened to go to the bathroom.

The drive home was far more pleasant. We both fell into bed exhausted, our three-hour excursion on this particular section of the Oncology Adventure Ride now complete. I hung the urine collection bag on the bed rail and remembered nothing else as sleep enveloped consciousness.

The official diagnosis written on the ER discharge instructions was "urinary retention." Those two words conveyed neither the mental panic of being unable to pee, nor the exquisite torment of an ever-filling bladder that lacked an exit. After awaking the next morning, I called Gail, the head nurse at Rad Onc and recounted the previous night's adventure. "I'll be sure to set up an appointment for you with Dr. Massullo and let Shari and Gretchen know you've got a catheter," she responded with friendly professionalism.

Just after crawling up on the narrow treatment table for the last time, and as Shari and Gretchen were adjusting my position with their usual tugs and nudges, a friendly voice rang out, "Now who was that guy who assured you just two days ago that no strictures would occur?" Dr. Massullo entered the treatment room with a wide yet sympathetic grin. His self-deprecating humor was exactly what the doctor ordered. "I think you should keep the Foley in for the next four or five days, but now that radiation is ending, it won't get any worse. Of course it can't," he added, still smiling.

The last session under the Novalis was as unremarkable as all sixteen that had preceded it—and the twenty-five under the Primus that preceded those. At last, there were no more days to count down. Gretchen and Shari both entered the room. Shari lowered the table and I hopped off. "Congratulations, Craig," Gretchen smiled as Shari handed me a "Certificate of Completion" signed by the staff people I'd come to know so well over the past nine weeks. Both gave me a hug and we wished each other good luck. It was over. My long march through radiotherapy was complete. In addition to the suitable-for-framing certificate, I walked out of the Radiation Oncology Center with tangible souvenirs of the journey: proctitis, urethritis, a Foley catheter and 79 Grays of cumulative radiation, equivalent to almost 57,000 chest X-rays.*

COMBAT RIBBONS

As a junior officer in the United States Navy in the early 1970s, my uniform sported two colorful military ribbons. One of them was the National Defense Service Medal—sometimes derisively called the "Alive in '65" ribbon because it was issued to everyone on active duty in the US military. The other was the more significant Navy Achievement Medal, awarded to me by my first commanding officer. However, having never served in Vietnam, I hadn't earned any ribbons for actual combat. But now, having endured a rather different form of combat—forty-two sessions of radiotherapy and the ongoing march of hormone therapy—I felt I'd finally earned a combat ribbon to mark my long campaign through cancerland.

We now live in the age of "awareness ribbons" available for every conceivable disease and cause. Designed to be worn on a blouse or lapel, they are a narrow piece of ribbon formed into a single loop, taking on a vaguely anthropomorphic shape consisting of a "head"—the loop—above the two "legs" of the ribbon's open ends pointing downward. Together with the ribbons, colored silicone wristbands have taken on the same meaning.

Some believe that awareness ribbons and wristbands for cancer and other diseases trace their origin back to the yellow ribbons that were tied around trees during the Iranian hostage crisis of 1979–1980. But it was Jeremy Irons's appearance at the 1991 Tony Awards wearing a bright red satin loop in the lapel of his tuxedo that really launched the present age of awareness ribbons. Two AIDS advocacy groups, Broadway Cares/Equity Fights AIDS and Visual AIDS, wished to raise AIDS awareness in the show business community. Looking for a simple yet memorable symbol, they contracted with Amster Novelties of Queens, New York—a supplier of display and promotional items for cosmetic

---

*Over the course of forty-two radiotherapy sessions, I received a total radiation dose of 79,000 milliGrays. The average chest X-ray is about 1.4 milliGrays.

companies—to produce what that company called the "No. 3 satin loop." The advocacy groups decided the ribbon should be bright red. Not only did it symbolize the fight against AIDS—red for passion, for anger, for love—it also looked great on TV. Given the controversial nature of AIDS advocacy—this was the early 1990s—TV viewers were not told what the ribbon stood for. But the sight of the ribbon was so visually arresting that even in that era before the web, social media, and viral videos, the country quickly learned its meaning.

It didn't take long for advocates of other causes to realize that these little colored loops were a simple, highly visible, and non-threatening way to communicate solidarity with a specific cause. Entire websites are devoted to the promotion and sale of ribbons and wristbands in the whole spectrum of advocacy colors. Among the cancers: dark blue for colon cancer, purple for pancreatic cancer, maroon for multiple myeloma, pearl for lung cancer, and so on. The Lance Armstrong Foundation has been the main force behind the popularity of silicone wristbands as the alternative to the lapel ribbons. The Foundation's bright yellow wristbands embossed with "LiveStrong" have become the omnipresent symbol of the battle against cancer in general.

Shortly after receiving my radiation diploma, I visited the Prostate Cancer Foundation website (www.pcf.org) and ordered a package of wristbands of the light blue color that represents prostate cancer. I consider this wristband to be my combat ribbon, and I've been wearing it ever since. Not many people have asked me about it, though. Those few who do are invariably surprised when I tell them light blue represents prostate cancer.

But everyone knows what pink stands for.

I SEE THE PINK RIBBONS: A BRIEF HISTORY OF BREAST CANCER ADVOCACY

Each October, breast cancer awareness month, a stunning array of objects turns pink: Yoplait yogurt lids, Duracell batteries, KitchenAid mixers, Logitech computer mice, and a host of other consumer products. In the middle of the month, the White House is illuminated in pink for an evening. Pink ribbons adorn numerous businesses and public spaces. The website of the Susan G. Komen

Foundation—founded in 1982 and now the largest and wealthiest breast cancer advocacy organization—lists almost two hundred corporate sponsors, including thirty-seven corporations which donate more than $1 million per year to be members of the exclusive "Million Dollar Council Elite." Restaurants promote breast cancer awareness with special offers during October. Blogger Matthew Oliphant launched a "Pink for October" campaign in 2008, asking the writers of blogs and people managing commercial websites to turn their web pages pink during October. One Sunday in October sees players of that bastion of masculinity—the NFL—sporting pink ribbons on helmets, wristbands, and shoes. It's difficult to miss the underlying message: Pink is the color of the fight against breast cancer.

Pink's ubiquity leaves the strong impression that breast cancer is the number one killer of women. It isn't. Heart disease is. Breast cancer is not even the number one killer of women in the US among cancers. Lung cancer is.

The breast cancer awareness campaign has been so successful that advocates for other diseases, especially other cancers, can only look on in awe—and with more than a little envy. However, the road to "all things pink" has been a long one, and has taken enormous effort on the part of hundreds of thousands of women. There's much that advocates for other cancers can learn from the experience of the women and organizations behind the pink. Especially advocates for increased prostate cancer awareness, who emphasize the numerical similarities of the two diseases with the analogy, "Prostate cancer is to men as breast cancer is to women."

If we were seeking a precise date for the origin of the breast cancer advocacy movement, September 28, 1974, would be a good one. On this day, Betty Ford, then First Lady, underwent a mastectomy—and spoke publicly about it. Up to this time, breast cancer, if discussed at all, fell into the euphemistic category of "female problems." From today's perspective, the older treatment model for the disease seems almost barbaric. When breast cancer was suspected, the woman would report to the hospital, be anesthetized, and a biopsy performed by the surgeon. The biopsy would be quickly evaluated, and if cancerous cells were present, the surgeon would immediately perform the aggressive Halstead mastectomy, removing the entire breast, including muscle tissue and lymph nodes—all while the patient remained unconscious. Initial breast cancer advocacy efforts focused on separating the biopsy from the surgery, requiring informed consent from the patient herself before a breast could be removed. These efforts were successful, and the Halsted procedure was finally abandoned in the 1980s.

In 1985, Zeneca Pharmaceuticals (now AstraZeneca), the company that manufactures the breast cancer drugs Arimidex® and tamoxifen, founded the National Breast Cancer Awareness Month (NBCAM), to be held each October. While corporate self-interest was certainly at work—there were all those breast cancer drugs to sell, after all—the move to raise awareness tapped into a deep yearning that patients, their loved ones, and women had to take action against this widespread cancer.

In October 1983, "The Race for the Cure" was held for the first time in Dallas, Texas. Eight hundred runners participated, raising money for breast cancer research. In recent years, the total number of participants in these races has exceeded 1.5 million, and the event has been held in over 100 U.S. cities, as well as in Canada, Australia, and several European countries.

In the 25 years since the creation of NBCAM, the number of organizations and businesses supporting the event has grown almost exponentially. In the fall of 1991, the Susan G. Komen Foundation handed out pink ribbons—shaped in the now-familiar single loop—to breast cancer survivors at a New York City road race. Two years later, the Senior Vice President of the Estee Lauder Companies, Evelyn Lauder, founded the Breast Cancer Research Foundation and took the pink ribbon as its logo. By the twenty-fifth anniversary of NBCAM, pink seemed to be flying everywhere in testimony to the most successful awareness-raising campaign in American history.

However, for those advocating greater awareness of prostate cancer and looking to breast cancer advocacy as a model, there is a cautionary side to this success story. Widespread corporate participation—and the desire to link brands to a noble cause that also demonstrates the company's commitment to gender equity—has come at a cost. Some advocates worry that the tight links between breast cancer and corporate messaging has compromised the movement's original goals. Since most breast cancer survivors tend to be white, well-educated, and middle- to upper-middle class, other advocates have taken the darker view that companies have joined the cause primarily to increase sales and profits in this highly-desirable demographic. In 2001, the Avon Foundation, sponsor of the Three Day Walk, was challenged by a coalition of breast cancer and women's health organizations for a lack of accountability in where funds raised by the walks were distributed.

There is even a phenomenon of over-awareness. In a 2001 article about her experience with breast cancer, author Barbara Ehrenreich hinted that the pinkness might be overtaking the disease, as she described

> ... a cornucopia of pink-ribbon-themed breast-cancer products. You can dress in pink-beribboned sweatshirts, denim shirts, pajamas, lingerie, aprons, loungewear, shoelaces, and socks; accessorize with pink rhinestone brooches, angel pins, scarves, caps, earrings, and bracelets; brighten up your home with breast-cancer candles, stained-glass pink-ribbon candleholders, coffee mugs, pendants, wind chimes, and night-lights; pay your bills with special BreastChecks or a separate line of Checks for the Cure.

Even so, there is more than corporate marketing wrapped in actual or apparent altruism at work here—and here is where the useful lesson for effective prostate cancer advocacy might be. An essential and powerful component behind the "pink explosion" has been the battalions of survivors and their loved ones intent not only on raising awareness and providing screening, but on increasing government funding for cancer research. The energy behind this drive has come from hundreds of smaller organizations, which the authors of *Cancer Activism* call grassroots survivor organizations (GSOs).

In the years following the creation of National Breast Cancer Awareness Month, grassroots advocacy groups designed to empower women—with or without breast cancer—sprang up all over the country. Most of these groups began with the mission to educate patients about their breast cancer treatment options. It was not long, however, until many of these groups turned to more political goals. As the authors of *Cancer Activism* observe,

An unusual convergence of events led to the development of breast cancer advocacy groups. First, many of the women who began to develop breast cancer in the late 1980s and early 1990s were well-educated, politically skilled, and had been involved in the civil rights and feminist movements. They considered breast cancer as another way to move from the "personal" to the "political"—the hallmark of the American contemporary women's movement.

In 1991, many of these local groups came together to form the National Breast Cancer Coalition (NBCC). With goals that included promoting research into the causes of breast cancer and increasing involvement of breast cancer patients in advocacy, the NBCC had a membership of over six hundred organizations and seventy thousand individual members by 2008.

It's difficult to exaggerate the impact of this grassroots energy that has been masterfully coordinated and targeted by the NBCC at influential policy makers. Writing in the *New England Journal of Medicine* in 1997, Suzanne Fletcher of Harvard Medical School opined that activism had resulted in widespread screening for women aged 40 to 49, riding roughshod over medical wisdom. She warned that medical policy would be made

... in the halls of Congress, and on the front page of the New York Times, *or as a lead story on ABC's* World News Tonight. *... Whereas anecdotes constitute weak evidence in medical science, personal stories are powerful persuaders in a Senate hearing.*

The lobbying of Congress by NBCC-affiliated grassroots organizations resulted in the creation of the Congressionally Directed Medical Research Program (CDMRP) in 1992. Administered by the Department of Defense and independent of the National Institutes of Health and its National Cancer Institute, the CDMRP receives annual funding directly from Congress. Its mission is to award research grants aimed specifically at prevention, control, and cure. In keeping with its origins in advocacy, the CDMRP includes "consumer reviewers"—men and women who actually have the disease in question—on the scientific peer review panels that recommend which grant requests should be approved. The idea is to keep the awards focused on those research projects most likely to result in near-term benefit for patients. While breast cancer was the initial recipient of funding, the CDMRP has expanded to encompass research grants for a variety of diseases, including prostate cancer, and has awarded over $5 billion in grants since its inception. Thus, prostate cancer research has benefited tangibly from the grassroots efforts undertaken by breast cancer advocates.

BUT WHERE ARE THE LIGHT BLUE RIBBONS?

The number of new diagnoses of breast cancer and prostate cancer made each year in the US is eerily similar. The NCI estimates that 230,480 new cases of breast cancer in women and 240,890 new cases of prostate cancer were diagnosed in 2011. Prostate cancer has a slightly lower mortality rate per diagnosis than breast cancer: 39,520 women died of breast cancer in 2011 while 33,720 men died from prostate cancer. A woman has a one in seven chance of contracting breast cancer in her lifetime; a man has a one in six chance of developing prostate cancer. So, each year when the President declares September as National Prostate Cancer Awareness Month the question is, why don't we see blue ribbons in September with the ubiquity that we see pink ones in October? And why is the White House lit in pink for an evening in October but has never been illuminated in blue in September—or any other month?

The answers to these questions are complex. Certainly the most significant event in the recent history of prostate cancer diagnosis has been the widespread adoption of the PSA test, which has allowed cancers of the prostate to be detected at much earlier stages. Prior to the PSA test, most prostate cancer cases were diagnosed only after the disease was locally advanced or worse, had already metastasized. As the PSA test has become widely adopted, the number of early stage prostate cancer diagnoses has increased dramatically, as has the need for better information about treatment options and patient care. The downside is that early detection has led to overtreatment (although there is wide disagreement as to how much). Since the majority of prostate cancers are slow growing, aggressive treatments such as prostatectomy or radiotherapy can too often result in medical outcomes worse than the consequences of untreated but often slow-growing cancer.

Several patient support groups emerged in the 1980s: The American Prostate Society, Patient Advocates for Advanced Cancer Treatment (PAACT), and the Prostate Cancer (later changed to "Conditions") Education Council (PCEC), all which attempted to educate men about the screening tools and treatment options available to them. In 1989, the PCEC began offering free screenings—PSA tests and digital rectal exams during one week in September, which the organization dubbed "Prostate Cancer Awareness Week." In 1990, Us TOO International was founded in Chicago by five prostate cancer survivors, and now has more than 300 chapters in the US and other countries providing support, education, and awareness on a local level. In 1993, venture capitalist and financier Michael Milkin, a survivor of advanced prostate cancer, founded CaP CURE, now the Prostate Cancer Foundation (PCF), the largest non-governmental organization funding prostate cancer research.

While Betty Ford went public about her breast cancer in 1974, a similar inauguration of the prostate cancer awareness movement did not occur until 1991, when former U.S. Senator and 1996 presidential nominee Bob Dole announced he had been diagnosed with prostate cancer. Unlike other famous men who had faced the same disease, Dole decided to go public with the story of his diagnosis and treatment, and the challenges of living as a prostate cancer survivor, including publicly uttering the "I" words—impotence and incontinence.

In 1996, CaP CURE, Us TOO, the Men's Health Network, the American Prostate Society, and the American Urological Association formed an umbrella advocacy organization, the National Prostate Cancer Coalition (NPCC). Modeled on the NBCC, its mission was to increase government funding for prostate cancer research. However, unlike its breast cancer counterpart, which is comprised of hundreds of grassroots groups, the NPCC grassroots network is considerably smaller. In some ways, the organizational contrast of these two coalitions parallels sociological differences between women and men. As observed earlier, women tend to be more familiar and comfortable with networking and one-on-one communication, which leads naturally to grassroots organizing. On the other hand, men have tended to organize themselves in hierarchies across the ages: think regiment-battalion-company-platoon-squad. Hierarchies are effective in carrying out orders from higher levels, but they do not necessarily encourage spontaneity, consensus building, or influencing policy from the bottom up.

Intrinsic differences between the causes—and the sexes—also reflect themselves in the types of activities used to raise awareness of the respective cancers. While breast cancer advocates walk, run, race, ride, or even mountain climb, the *Cancer Activism* authors observe that "prostate cancer activities are much more passive: a mobile screening van or watching a sports event such as major league baseball or professional golf." The prostate cancer advocacy movement was also hindered in its early years, by turf battles at the organizational level. Us TOO resigned from the NPCC in 2001, stating it desired to return to its original local support mission. Others have criticized the Prostate Cancer Foundation for not participating actively in the NPCC.

By 2008, there was growing recognition that disparate, uncoordinated advocacy organizations were not an effective way to advance awareness, and more importantly, to increase research funding. This awareness led twelve non-profit prostate cancer advocacy and research organizations to form the Prostate Cancer Roundtable in an effort to speak with a unified voice in public policy and awareness-building forums. A primary mission is raising Congressional appropriations for the CDMRP's Prostate Cancer Research Program, which is funded at less than half the level of the CDMRP's Breast Cancer Research Program. Longer-term goals include establishing an Office of Men's Health within the Department of Health and Human Services that would have a mission similar to that of the Office of Women's Health that has been operational since 1991.

As necessary and desirable as these advocacy organizations are, and as encouraging as it is that they are beginning to work together, building national awareness of prostate cancer with a similar level of success achieved by breast cancer movement has not yet occurred. Gender-related cancer advocacy is one area where traditional male dominance and glass ceilings do not apply. While the prostate cancer advocacy movement is

Member Organizations of the Prostate Cancer Roundtable

Ed Randall's Fans for the Cure (www.fansforthecure.org)

Malecare (malecare.org)

Men's Health Network (www.menshealthnetwork.org)

National Alliance of State Prostate Cancer Coalitions (www.naspcc.org)

Prostate Cancer Foundation (www.pcf.org)

Prostate Cancer International (pcainternational.org)

Prostate Conditions Education Council (www.prostateconditions.org)

The Prostate Health Education Network (www.prostatehealthed.org)

The Prostate Net (www.prostate-online.com)

Us TOO International Prostate Cancer Education and Support Network (www.ustoo.org)

Women Against Prostate Cancer (www.womenagainstprostatecancer.org)

ZERO – The Project to End Prostate Cancer (zerocancer.org)

well aware of—and often imitates breast cancer advocacy strategies—the converse is not true. Some breast cancer advocates are not even aware that a prostate cancer advocacy movement exists.

Finally, there are intrinsic behavioral differences between the sexes. As noted earlier, men are often reluctant to speak openly with others about their bodies, much less about a disease that that attacks them at the nexus of their sexual identity. In 2003, the former president of Us TOO stated,

> *We're in the 1985 range of where breast cancer was. A lot of men don't want to talk about prostate cancer, much less come out and say, "I've had prostate cancer."*

In the end, it is this reticence—especially when contrasted with the relative willingness of women to talk freely about breast cancer—that hinders greater awareness. Less advocacy has important consequences: not only are there fewer light blue ribbons than pink ones, but more crucially, there is less funding directed toward finding a cure.

WHERE THE MONEY GOES

Since Richard Nixon declared the "War on Cancer" with the passage of the 1971 National Cancer Act, the National Cancer Institute (NCI) has expended billions of dollars to attack the disease on many fronts. A former director of the NCI asserted in 2005 that

> *"[the NCI] did everything it was supposed to do. It supported basic research handsomely. It set up application programs ... and U.S. clinical trials programs. The incidence of cancer in this country started dropping in 1990 and has continued to drop every year since, and so has mortality. And the morbidity from cancer, comparing 1971 to 2005, is like night and day.... So, every benchmark of the [war on cancer] mandate has been hit."*

This optimistic statement notwithstanding, definitive cures for virtually every type of cancer still lie in the future.

While significant sums for cancer research are also spent by private organizations such as the American Lung Association, the Susan G. Komen Foundation, and the Prostate Cancer Foundation to identify causes of and treatments for lung, breast and prostate cancer, respectively, the federal government provides the majority of the research funds. Unsurprisingly, the National Cancer Institute has the biggest share of government funding approximately $5.25 billion in 2011, although other federal government departments spend money on cancer research as well, most notably the Department of Defense via the CDMRP described earlier.

Of course, not all cancers receive an equal share of research dollars. While there are numerous factors that influence Congress, there can be little doubt that the success of breast cancer advocates had led to more money being allocated to breast cancer research than to any other cancer.

In 2011, lung cancer diagnoses totaled an estimated 221,130 new cases in the US. Statistically, it is the most lethal cancer, with almost 157,000 estimated deaths in the same year. In 2008 (a typical year, since overall cancer funding has remained relatively flat for several years), the NCI spent $572.6 million on breast cancer research, or about $3100 per newly diagnosed case. NCI-funded prostate cancer research for the same year was $285.4 million, a little more than $1500 per newly diagnosed case. But before men with prostate cancer begin complaining about their second-class status, consider lung cancer: 2008 NCI funding of $247.6 million works out to about $1150 per newly diagnosed case of a disease with a far higher mortality rate than either breast or prostate cancer.

More starkly, if we view the amounts that the NCI spends on a "per cancer death basis," breast cancer expenditures (about $14,000 per death) still ranks number one. Prostate cancer, because of its slightly lower mortality rate compared to breast cancer, comes in second at about $10,000 spent per death. But when compared to lung cancer at a mere $1,530 per death, the disparity is dramatic. As Tara Parker-Hope, writing in the *New York Times* health blog, points out,

> *The big loser in the cancer funding race is lung cancer. It is the biggest cancer killer in the country, yet on a per-death basis receives the least NCI funding among major cancers.*

Of course many variables affect the funding equation, including the public perception of a particular cancer. As we have seen, advocates for breast cancer research have been highly effective influencing NCI's and the CDMRP's ultimate funding source: Congress. Also, both lung and prostate cancer tend to be "old person's diseases," while breast cancer—especially its more aggressive forms—often strikes young, otherwise healthy women. Lung cancer's public image is further tarnished by the widespread belief that the lung cancer patient is probably responsible for contracting his disease from years of smoking. This rationale provides little comfort to lung cancer patients who never smoked.

Perhaps there are even more fundamental psychological issues at work here. All of us fed at, or were at least held close to, our mother's breasts as babies. One writer commenting at the *New York Times* health blog stated,

> [Breast cancer's high funding level] is related to a fundamental way in which we identify women—in which women identify themselves, and in which men and children feel about them. Everyone has strong primal feelings about breasts. It's just not the same with any other part of the human body. With that primal underpinning, breast cancer research becomes an unassailable brand. . . .

Men and women rarely use the same strategy to accomplish a particular goal. Prostate cancer advocates can employ many of the techniques that have worked to advance awareness and advocacy for breast cancer, but there is no point in simply copying them. Being a disease diagnosed primarily in men over the age of 65, prostate cancer advocacy faces a generational reality: Up until now, most diagnosed men have been members of the Greatest Generation or the Korean War generation. As we have seen, these cohorts tend to endure illness in stoic silence. But as the comparatively more self-aware (and self-centered) baby boom generation ages, its male members will comprise the majority of prostate cancer patients within the next few years. Given the boomer generation's proclivity for activism, it's a reasonably safe prediction that prostate cancer finally will begin to share center stage with breast cancer. The light blue ribbons will become more widely recognized as men become increasingly willing to speak of a formerly "unspeakable" disease.

Amidst the cultural mores, organizational battles, and all these numbers and dollars, we are compelled to remember one central point: advocacy, media attention, and policy initiatives are all a positive force. Too many men and women still die from cancer each year. The War on Cancer may be a tired metaphor, but cancer's ubiquity means that the strategies, tactics, and individual skirmishes in the world of cancer awareness, advocacy, and funding remain crucially important to the health of American society at large.

PART IV
A LIFETIME'S JOURNEY

TEN

OK, God, So Where Are You, Anyway?

COMMUNITY MATTERS

It's always more fun when friends ride a roller coaster together. Because they share the experience, screaming in unison at steep descents and sharp turns, the ride somehow seems less terrifying. At some subconscious level, people probably believe that sticking together as a group makes it more likely that they'll come out the other side unscathed. Unfortunately, the Oncology Adventure Ride accommodates only a single rider. My wife, children, extended family, fellow cancer survivors, and friends all provided invaluable support, but they had to do it from the ride's platform. The biopsies, injections, hot flashes, radiation treatments, and, above all, the feelings and reflections brought on by this disease were mine to experience alone.

Given my personality, I should have been quite happy in my solitude. I am an introvert who has learned some extroverted skills such as public speaking and cocktail party chit chat, but I have never felt at ease in a crowd, especially a crowd that was suddenly being so solicitous of its cancer-stricken friend. I was raised to believe that too much personal attention led to pride. So, as long as I can remember, I skillfully deployed sarcasm and self-deprecating humor to keep intimacy at arm's length.

But now something was changing. My strategy was starting to unravel. Why should a cancer diagnosis alter a life philosophy that had worked so well for almost sixty years? I wasn't sure. But somehow it had. I only knew that, where I once felt confidence, I now felt loneliness, even abandonment.

When my wife Susan first suggested that, during my course of radiation, we might want to meet regularly with some close friends to talk and pray, my initial (and carefully unspoken) reaction was unenthusiastic at best. "Great. It's not enough to endure the joys of living without testosterone and undergoing radiation along with a daily fifty-two-mile commute," I thought silently. "Let's add intimate social interaction to the schedule." But as I reflected on her suggestion, my initial resentment faded. Perhaps getting together with people I knew well would ameliorate that uneasy feeling that something significant and scary was indeed happening to me. Unlike the side effects of ADT and radiation, praying would certainly do no physical harm, and it might even do some psychological and spiritual good.

With a few phone calls, Susan had it all set up. We'd meet at the house of one of the couples that had volunteered to be members of our little band. And so—as translators of the King James Bible might have phrased it—it came to pass that four couples gathered every Wednesday afternoon following my radiotherapy session to converse and to pray for each other. We had all known each other for years, which allowed the conversation to be open and honest. What evolved was eight weeks of authentic sharing, as each person spoke in turn—about adult children, financial issues, or other health concerns. In so doing, the focus of the group extended far beyond just "Craig's cancer." I was an equal partner in a journey being taken together. While others were praying for me, I could pray for them. This equality helped to keep any tendency toward self-pity in check and to restore some equilibrium during a time that felt so off-balance in almost every other way.

Several people have asked me why I never joined a cancer support group during this time. This small group was the reason why. In the sanctity and safety of these seven other men and women, two of whom were themselves cancer survivors, I found my community of support that made this phase of my journey not only bearable, but comforting.

For many years I've been meeting with a group of other men on Friday mornings for breakfast. Along with eggs, oatmeal, and coffee, we study—dissect would be the more accurate word—the 100-year-old, but still completely relevant, devotional writings of Oswald Chambers. One morning, a couple of weeks after radiotherapy had begun, one of these men, Smit, pulled a small plastic bag from his pocket. As he opened it he said, "Last week I was down in Mexico with our high school youth as we worked on building houses down there. Each night when I lay down on my sleeping bag to pray, I could think of only one person: Craig. So I brought these." He handed each man at the table, including me, a Kelly green silicone wristband etched with the words, "Pynn your prayers on Craig." In my pre-cancer life I would have objected (probably with typically sarcastic humor) to the use of my last name as a verb and a pun. But this morning I was speechless as each man around the table put on the wristband and promised to wear it until my radiation course was complete. No cancer support group could have provided more meaningful encouragement than that simple, generous gesture.

The willingness of my family and close friends to stick by me through the ups, downs, twists, and turns of the Oncology Adventure Ride was how I came to believe that something spiritually profound was happening alongside my clinical encounter with cancer. I may have been on this metaphorical roller coaster ride alone, but I was not alone in the real world. Witnessing how a caring community stood so close to me in my journey helped me realize that my lifelong practice of going it alone was an ego-based delusion. All those accomplishments I always thought were uniquely mine had been possible only because other people were always nearby and cared about me.

Mark Nepo is a poet and philosopher—and a cancer survivor. He writes how the creation of a support community can have a life-altering impact on each member, regardless of who actually has the disease:

> *Sharing pain is the only way to stay alive. For the net of love helps absorb and distribute the struggle. It's taught me that if we share pain, which is a lot to ask, there is no room*

for pity. For the sharing of the struggle requires an invest-
ment, a real life-changing investment by those who care,
an involvement that will instigate their own tandem suf-
fering … We are well today, because those who love us got
involved, deeply involved, daily involved. And by being so
healed, we are forever wed to their pain. We are forever open
to their struggles. By being so loved, we can never shut our
lives again.

I had so valued the supposed merits of rugged individual-
ism that I had forgotten how dependent each of us actually
is—and must always remain—on each other. So, in its process
of upsetting my self-centered equilibrium, my cancer had
opened me to seeing what others have long known: Sharing
each other's joys and struggles is how we grow and mature as
individuals. My support community stuck close by not because
they felt duty bound, but because they honestly wanted to ease
my suffering, to lighten my burden. And, yes, because they
loved me.

These experiences as a member of a genuine caring community taught me that my experience with cancer was much more
than a solo excursion on the Oncology Adventure Ride. Those
who stood by my side had—knowingly or not—joined me on an
expedition of the soul.

THE PARALLEL JOURNEY

Hearing the words "You have a nasty prostate cancer" (or any
kind of cancer) rattles the soul as much as the body. Maybe that
simultaneous assault on the physical and the spiritual is one of
the things that make cancer a dreaded disease. For me, hearing
those words had a visceral impact not unlike the feeling one
gets in last few seconds before passing out. As Dr. Hopkins told
me the news, my surroundings blurred into gray indistinct-
ness, and I felt as if I were falling headfirst into a chasm that
lay beyond ordinary space and time. Falling alongside me into
this void was my belief that I was firmly in control of just about
every aspect of my existence, including the assurance of a long
and healthy life. In those rare moments when I actually thought

about it, I had seen my future covering boundless stretches of time that seemed to be my rightful allotment. After all, I was a relatively young 62 years old. I had envisioned spending my remaining years fulfilling my lengthy checklist of Things in Life Yet to Be Accomplished. This was no "bucket list." It included continued productive labor, perhaps adding in some volunteer work, as well as many more cross-country trips between California and Massachusetts with Susan. I would watch my grandchildren grow, mature, graduate from high school and college, and perhaps even see them have children of their own. (After all, my own father had already enjoyed all these experiences.) And one day, when things settled down, I would study theology more seriously, perhaps learn some Koine Greek. Or, perhaps I would finally write that book … on high technology marketing.

The idea that some intrusive disease could possibly cut short my entitled allocation of years had simply never entered my head. I was a baby boomer after all, and we boomers have always embraced visions of immortality. But as the shadow of my vulnerability loomed in Dr. Hopkins's office on that cold January morning, I knew in my gut that the cancer was real—and that it was going to change a lot of things, not the least of which were my smug assumptions about being in control. Perceiving one's mortality is not the same as fearing death. In my case, it was realizing that my rock-solid assumptions about my future life were not rock-solid after all: that I wouldn't live indefinitely, that I had infinitely less power over my personal fate than I had thought.

This sense of being in control had been dramatically challenged only once before in my life. But I had been able to repair it quickly. Fifteen years before, in the trauma unit at John Muir Hospital, after arriving unconscious with a smashed face and broken ribs from an automobile accident, I awoke briefly. Just before blackness closed in again, I remember lying there, looking up into the faces of strangers working on parts of my body, wondering who they were and what they were doing—all without my instructions or assistance. Confined to a hospital bed over the next seven days, I had realized that believing I was firmly and constantly in control of my thoughts, actions—and future—was a delusion. On leaving the hospital, I had every intention of reminding myself frequently that while we humans are beautifully equipped to create the illusion of being in control, we should not fall for the trick. But even the most sincere resolutions have a habit of fading away as the body heals. By the time Dr. Hopkins told me I had "a nasty cancer," I had been residing comfortably in my fantasy of control for a long time.

Hearing your doctor tell you that you have cancer is different than arriving unconscious at an ER trauma unit. Nothing had changed physically; this time there was no smashed face or broken ribs. I had walked into Dr. Hopkins's office with the cancer; it hadn't just materialized at his pronouncement of the words, "You have aggressive cancer." It had been growing stealthily inside me for some time—at least several months, perhaps several years already. Physically, I looked the same after hearing his words. Even when the hematuria had occurred a few months before, there had been no pain, and I had felt none since then. Only the raw intellectual knowledge that I had cancer was new. But that single piece of information instantly connected itself to all the other data that I'd acquired over the years. Faces of the people I once knew—now dead from cancer—including Ron Borrelli passed before my mind's eye.

It was at this moment that fear stepped into the room and stood silently behind me. Not so much the fear of dying (that would come later), but a more persistent worry that I was somehow no longer a whole person. I vaguely sensed that cancer had carved something important out of my being. Swinging hard from serene self-confidence, I now could only see myself as a shell: a simulacrum of the real Craig Pynn.

Everything was the same; everything was completely different. This feeling of carved-outness, of what I came to call *not-wholeness*, became increasingly palpable over the days and weeks following the diagnosis. This was not just a fear of what might happen to me physically, although that fear was real enough. Something else, not just cancer, was gnawing at my innards. Carefully arranged mental furniture had been knocked about into a jumble of anxiety and doubt. And one other thing had become obvious in the midst of this foreboding: God was certainly no longer smiling on me.

Looking back, I see that a significant spiritual journey paralleling the medical one began that morning in the exam room at Pacific Urology. As the clinical path moved inexorably from diagnosis to treatment decisions, so too the spiritual trek moved from the illusion of self-sufficiency to new vistas that would not have revealed themselves had I never been diagnosed with cancer. I now see how this spiritual journey has forced me to reexamine my fundamental assumptions about what Douglas Adams, author of *Hitchhiker's Guide to the Galaxy*, so aptly termed, "life, the universe, and everything." But before my quest could really begin in earnest, a big question still had to be confronted: Why me?

IT'S JUST NOT FAIR

Like many Americans, I have a culturally inbred sense of fairness. It's an axiom: Despite whatever tribulations that may occur along the way, in the end, the good guys are supposed to win; the bad guys are supposed to lose. This logic holds in popular fiction, movies, and modern myths, like Star Wars and Harry Potter. When fictional characters contract a life-threatening disease like cancer, they can certainly suffer, but after many trials, they eventually triumph, spiritually, if not physically. Bad people contracting some dread illness always pay a high price—dying does nicely—unless they repent just before the end credits roll. Our stories often reflect how our culture wants things to be. But of course, the real world doesn't work that neatly. Good people get cancer—and many die from it.

I had paid close attention to the state of my prostate by dint of annual DREs and PSA tests over the past ten years in an effort to avoid what had just happened. The unfairness-of-it-all hobgoblin loomed large, especially in the dark, quiet hours before dawn, immediately following that brief interval between returning to consciousness and remembering that I had cancer. Then one day I came across a story that dealt with serious unfairness that put my own plight in its proper perspective.

Already dealing with chronic pain in his legs, William Stuntz, a professor at Harvard Law School, was diagnosed with colon cancer and experienced all the ugly side effects of chemotherapy. He states bluntly, "Cancer will very probably kill me within the next two years. I'm 50 years old." Stuntz realizes that life is unfairly random, observing,

Though I deserve every bad thing that has happened to me, those things didn't happen because I deserve them. Life in a fallen world is more arbitrary than that. Plenty of people deserve a better life than I do, but get much worse. Some deserve worse and get much better.

Clearly, Stuntz has thought long and hard about the question of fairness:

The question we are most prone to ask when hardship strikes—why me?—makes no sense. That question presupposes that pain, disease, and death are distributed according to moral merit. They aren't. We live in a world in which innocent children starve while moral monsters prosper. We may see justice in the next life, but we see little of it in this one.

The answer to the question "Why me?" seems to be that life in the here and now is manifestly unfair. In 1987, I witnessed this unfairness first hand when my best friend, Steve, died of complications arising from AIDS. This was shortly after AIDS had been identified as a disease, and little about it was yet understood from a scientific perspective—and even less from a sociological one. A popular TV preacher claimed the scourge was God's revenge on homosexual sin. It would be difficult to imagine a life more honestly and decently lived than Steve's. He and his wife Linda were adoptive parents of five young children. Steve had been on kidney dialysis for many years due to an adolescent bout with nephritis. Having waited years for a kidney transplant, he finally received a call from a hospital in San Francisco in early 1981 that a matching kidney had become available. At first, the operation appeared to be a success. But then his postoperative course deteriorated, and Steve endured severe flu-like symptoms. For reasons the doctors did not really understand, Steve's body rejected the kidney a week after the transplant, and it was removed in a second operation. Within two months, he was diagnosed with what we now know to be HIV. In acts of breathtaking arrogance, some devout but thoroughly misguided acquaintances of Steve's, clothed in religious self-righteousness, told him that he must have committed some grievous moral wrong to be afflicted so severely.

Those were the days before drug cocktails were able to hold full-blown AIDS at bay for many years. Linda, their children, and friends—including me—watched for six years as Steve slowly wasted away from the effects of a virus that no one at the time knew had been lurking in the blood transfusions he had received with the transplant. In July 1987, Steve died, a victim of life's profound unfairness.

That was when I came to know that disease and death are not, in Stuntz's words, "distributed according to moral merit." Giving the eulogy at Steve's memorial service was the moment I finally understood, "Yes, life is indeed unfair." But rather than reflecting further on what that unfairness might mean to me personally, I packaged "life is unfair," into a neat little mental box, and filed it away under "life's truths." There it sat pretty much undisturbed until I was diagnosed with cancer in early 2009.

When bad things happen to other people, even one's best friend, unfairness still tends to remain an abstraction: unfortunate, often tragic, but, hey, that's how life is. It's a reality we must accept philosophically: Bad stuff happens. But when cancer came to me personally, the blatant, arbitrary unfairness of life pushed a white-hot poker straight through my being as my dreams of a limitless future came crashing to earth. That compact little box of "life is unfair" fell off its mental shelf and tumbled open, spilling its ugly contents. "This can't be happening to me," I thought. "This is completely unjust. I've lived a clean, sober life; supported my family; raised our children. I've worked hard for many years and now just when it's time for some fun I get cancer? This sucks beyond imagination." Chaotic feelings jostled against each other with increasing energy, but at their center was the singularly clear sentence, "This is so damn unfair."

Ever a stoic, I said nothing about my feelings of unfairness to anyone, even to Susan. Too many physical and emotional challenges were already in play; there was no time to be brooding about the philosophical concept of unfairness. I swept up the shards of "this is so unfair" and stuffed them once again into their little box, setting it back on my mental shelf. However, the box remained undisturbed for only a few weeks when my brother-in-law, Nick, raised the unfairness issue in an email to me. Nick was an attorney, who became a paraplegic at the age of eighteen, so he was well experienced with life's unfairness. He wrote:

> *During my many years of therapy one of the themes I worked on ... was the perceived—rightly or wrongly—unfairness of life. For years, [my therapist] urged me to try and "enjoy" the difficulties in life.... [He told me that] all the difficulties do not go away, so it is best to incorporate them into life as it goes on. I struggled with this idea, and fought it. But eventually I began to understand, and now find that when times are tough I tend to go with the flow. So, I guess my advice is to find a way to enjoy the experience—not because it will be enjoyable, but because it is a part of life—your life—and you wouldn't want it to be anyone else's.*

Nick's advice seems right. There are really only two options when it comes to dealing with life's unfairness. One is to become an embittered victim. But as we've seen already, victimhood and its attendant resentment is a dead-end slide into despair. The second option, as Nick points out, is to integrate, however awkwardly, the unfairness into our daily lives and struggle forward.

But his conclusion, as wise as it was, still felt too existential. Wasn't there a larger purpose here than to simply and calmly realize that life unreels movie-like, and that the issue is not judging each event as good or bad, but simply accepting them "as is"? Just accept the cancer, Craig, and move on. But move on to where? Or did my cancer's unfairness have a larger lesson to teach me? Stoic acceptance is doubtless necessary, but it sure seemed like there needed to be something more. Thinking about unfairness only amplified my feeling of incompleteness, that gnawing *not-wholeness* that had materialized like a morning fog when I heard Dr. Hopkins's pronouncement. Accepting the intrinsic unfairness of life may have been necessary, but mere acceptance was not sufficient. Something more was definitely required.

IS THERE MORE THAN MERELY THIS?

"Is That All There Is?" is the title of a song made popular by the singer Peggy Lee in the late 1960s. Quintessentially representative

of that decade's angst, the song meditates on the many disillu-
sionments of life. But when I first heard that song in 1969, and
upon hearing it occasionally ever since, it seems to pose a meta-
physical big question in musical guise: What, if anything, exists
beyond our physical day-to-day reality? There's a continuum
of possible answers ranging from the materialist's "Nothing, of
course! There's only what can be scientifically demonstrated and
proven," to the declarations of the fervently religious, "God completely controls every aspect of His creation; after all, He knows
when even a sparrow falls."

Before my diagnosis, I came down courageously between
those extremes. My materialist side was expressed in the firm
belief in the primacy and efficacy of the laws of physics and evo-
lutionary biology. Simultaneously, on the spiritual side, I believed
in a transcendent God, who created everything that exists. Unlike
the deist, who believes God created the universe, set it in motion,
and then left it to unfold undisturbed, I believed that God continues to operate within His creation, not only through the laws
of physics and the rules of biology, but in the hearts and minds
of men and women. More importantly, I believe, He cares deeply
about His creation—and especially values us human beings,
lovingly created in His image. The apotheosis of God's creative
extravagance is His gift of a free will that allows us, among an
infinity of other choices, even to reject the whole idea of God.
Inexplicably (at least in human terms), God still loves us in spite
of the nefarious consequences—as amply demonstrated throughout history—arising from us humans enthusiastically exercising
our God-given free will.

There's nothing particularly original about my theology, and
even though I have believed in this Creator God since I was a
child, I have never heard a Voice, nor have I experienced one
of those ineffable moments that others describe where Christianity's claims became blindingly obvious or tangibly real. Ever
since I began reflecting seriously on spiritual matters as an adult,
I have always relied on my powers of reasoning to deduce my
way into belief. Religious people, including many Christians,
posit that feeling and emotion lie at the center of true belief—
what they call "belief of the heart"—implicitly relegating those
like me, who have valued reason above feeling to a less exalted
location, sometimes called "head belief" or "religion of the

mind." Even so, my belief in God's love and His presence in this world had become sufficiently persuasive to me that for more than thirty years I worked to demonstrate—looking back, I suppose it was mainly to myself—that my intellectually deduced belief system was just as valid as (if not occasionally superior to) the more emotional spiritual experiences of others. As the years progressed, I had become an active churchgoer, worshipped regularly, served on the church council, led Bible studies, and enjoyed the community of fellow believers, many of whom were my closest friends. To me, anyway, my faith seemed to be quite robust. Not surprisingly, this perception fit quite nicely with my sense of being in control, because I had arrived at this satisfying position pretty much on my own intellectual steam.

That is, until *notwholeness* crept in unbidden. The only metaphor I could summon for this feeling was a void, something like a small black hole inhabiting my otherwise complete self. Had cancer created this carved-out hollowness? Maybe. Or had it taken a personal crisis like this to force me to stare more honestly into a dark chasm that had been there all along? It didn't really matter. The question was not whether cancer had created the *notwholeness*, this lacuna of being. The critical issue was that cancer had exposed it.

Up to this point, I had a plethora of intellectual arguments to help me resist the claims of those who asserted that genuine belief also involved the heart—that storied seat of emotion. But now, with my sense of control wrested away, mental power and logical deduction were proving insufficient. However reluctantly, it was time to make the journey down from my head toward my heart. In order to honestly answer the question "Is that all there is?" I had to leave my walled city of intellect, with its proud towers of logic and deduction, and venture out into the dark and threatening landscape of the emotional and spiritual.

To pass the time waiting at various medical offices, I had been reading *Surprised by Hope* by N.T. Wright. Wright has a fresh take on Christian beliefs about death. Retrospectively, I see that this was a propitious moment to discover a theologian who employs logic and reason to elucidate matters of the heart.

Wright's declaration that heaven is not some vague, mystical and far away cloudland, a sort of eternal church service, but "the other, hidden, dimension of our ordinary life—God's dimension, if you like" struck me forcefully. As Wright says elsewhere,

[Heaven is not some] blissful disembodied life after death in which creation is abandoned to its fate, but rather the hope ... for the renewal and final coming together of heaven and earth, the consummation precisely of God's project to be savingly present in [the] world.

Wright's assertion that heaven and earth are congruent, and will become one united creation at the end of history was a bold new idea for me. Up to this point I had a bifurcated mental model of God's relationship to humankind: We were stuck here on earth, pretty much left to our own devices; God was transcendent—unfathomable and omnipotent—but He was somewhere else than right here. Yes, He was a loving God, but a loving distant God. And like most Christians, I figured that my ultimate heavenly reward lay somewhere off in a hazy but certainly happy future after we died. Up to this point, given my assumption about living a long, healthy life, I hadn't really given the subject of what happens when we're dead much thought at all. But what Wright calls "God's project" is that God wants us to be "a genuine human being contributing to God's project of justice and beauty ... bringing justice, hope, joy and beauty to God's world." Wright is saying firmly that our raison d'être for being here in the first place is to seek justice, promote beauty, and tell others about the good news in the right here and the right now. The phrase resonated: "right here and right now." As I absorbed Wright's assertion, I felt—instead of reasoned—that God was really much closer to me than I had assumed all these years. As the cliché has it, God was right next to me all the time.

This was hardly an original insight. There's a word for God's proximity: immanence. It comes from the Latin, meaning "to remain within" and it has a rich theological tradition, which lies beyond our discussion here. I interpret immanence to mean that God's unfathomable love encompasses—among other things—the four dimensions of space and time that we occupy, including our own right here and right now. God may be infinite and far beyond me, yet He is at once extraordinarily close at hand. Around the same time I was absorbing Wright's thesis, our Friday morning men's group came across a related statement by Oswald Chambers, rough the moments." That is: God's presence is not only tangible reality that can be experienced in real space and real time, it is in fact reality itself. These two men, writing one hundred years apart in time spoke the identical thought to me: God is much closer to you than you think, and He is reality. God is not an intellectual abstraction.

Perhaps it's natural for this kind of revelation to occur in times of personal trial, but looking back, I see how cancer has deepened my awareness of God's immanence. Even though I've often heard others speak about being close to their "personal God," it was a radical new idea for me. Maybe this was what all this heart business was about, I thought: It's the sensory organ that is tuned into God's reality.

Using this newly discovered sensory power of the heart, I began looking for evidence of God's closeness. He was surely there in the silence of the Rad Onc patient's waiting room. I could see God's love mysteriously reflected in the resigned, yet accepting faces of my companions there. These faces in which, after all the weeks of radiation and for many of them, also weeks and even months of chemotherapy, every social mask, every pretension had been stripped away. Instead, each face, in its transparent honesty seemed to mirror God's order of the moments, life as it truly is. And after a while, I realized while lying on the treatment table that I was not really so alone in the lead-lined room after all. The sense of peace amid the moving and buzzing machinery came from a God who had always been there.

My new awareness of God's immanence manifested itself in other ways. Lengthy prayers by others, which had always seemed so pointlessly verbose, took on new richness, and some even began to feel too brief.

To be clear: This has been my spiritual journey and, retrospectively, much that was opaque before now appears obvious ... to me. It's not unlike having the inner workings of a magic trick explained. My experience is assuredly not an instruction about how others should make their own journey. They may quite legitimately come to a completely different place that excludes God altogether. However, I submit that each person who takes the time to reflect—regardless of whether he or she has a disease like cancer—will discern that same sensation of *notwholeness* that I felt. And in that apparent nothingness, he or she is likely to encounter the ineffable. Cancer, or any other threatening illness or trauma, just happens to be extraordinarily efficient at wiping away the distractions we so carefully erect in order to mask those feelings of *notwholeness*.

THE PROBLEM OF PRAYERS FOR HEALING

As with human relationships—especially when they are put to the test by a disease like cancer—establishing and maintaining a thriving relationship with God must include honest communication, which by definition is a two-way affair: clear transmission and reception are required at both ends. People hear God speak in a variety of ways: studying the Bible; reading devotional works or the writings of the church fathers; through their labor or in their artistry; or simply by meditation. Others may see visions and hear voices. Of course a God who speaks to us through circumstances surely speaks to us through the words and deeds of those around us. Lutheran pastor Sara Wolbrecht observes that, "God will communicate with you in a way that corresponds with who you are."

As I've said, an intellectual approach to spiritual matters had long satisfied me, so my relationship with God over the years had come mainly through reading and studying the Bible, theological writings, listening to expository sermons and lectures, and above all, in small groups where people seriously discuss and wrestle with issues of faith. But when it comes to dealing with a life-altering disease such as cancer, there is one form of communication with an immanent God that is at once obvious, difficult, and even sometimes controversial: prayer. Prayer may be the most widely practiced means of speaking with God, but for me, it has always been the most uncomfortable. Prayer has seemed like God's cod liver oil: good for me, but hard to swallow.

A few days after hearing the scary words from Dr. Hopkins, I shared my diagnosis with the eight other people at my weekly men's group just before we adjourned. Thinking they would simply utter the usual sympathetic noises, and abstractly promise to pray for me, I was taken aback when, as we were walking out, one of the men named Kevin announced, "OK, guys, we need to pray for Craig right now." So, on the sidewalk of a busy street corner in Walnut Creek, California, eight men gathered around me, each placing a hand on my head or shoulder, as Kevin spoke an extemporaneous, heartfelt prayer explicitly asking God for my healing. This experience was simultaneously uplifting and anxiety producing. This was a generous, loving gesture that I would long treasure in my heart.

Yet, this event also created an uneasy feeling deep inside me. At first, I attributed this feeling to having been the unexpected center of attention of a group of men standing on a public street corner. But later, I realized that at least some portion of my discomfort arose from having never before been the object of a specific prayer for healing in quite so dramatic a fashion. Yes, people had prayed for my healing before, but it was always in a private setting, never on a public street. But there was something else going on here as well. What was it about this encounter besides its very public nature that made me so uneasy?

Reflecting on prayers for healing, I remembered that many of the people for whom I had prayed for healing had, in fact, been healed. Others, most notably my friend Steve, were not. Yes, life is unfair, and justice is unevenly distributed. Pete Apple, a retired Presbyterian pastor in Texas with advanced prostate cancer like mine, has struggled with this issue about how to pray for healing. He wrote to me in an email,

> It is both redundant and presumptuous to pray for God to heal [us]. It is redundant because the presence of God is a healing presence. It is presumptuous because it is "Give me what I want," assuming that this defines our relationship with God—because healing is God's job. Healing must be a gift of grace. Grace that is demanded is not grace [at all].

Pete is saying that it may be better to pray for the healing presence of God than for physical healing itself. This claim may be one that some people who pray may not accept.

The reality is that not everyone is healed—at least not with the physical healing we might prefer. And for me, therein lies the truth of prayers for healing, as it sheds fresh light on the problem of who gets healed and who doesn't. We are all healed one way or the other. This may or may not include physical healing, but regardless of our circumstances, a prayer of faith always results in being "raised up." This raising up may be spiritual, emotional, psychological, physical—or some combination of these. And when the faithful prayers of others surround us—as I was that winter morning—we will never fail to experience healing of the heart.

In the end, I must remember that regardless of how many prayers may have been said on my behalf, and no matter how much I wish it to be so, there is no guarantee I will be healed physically. As the owner of advanced cancer, however, I have become more comfortable with people praying for my healing. But I must always remember that it's not obvious what form my healing will take. Instead, it is better to think of it as a new healing each day.

Then there are my own prayers. My first prayer is to remember always that I am not the one in control here. The second prayer is for God to help me dismantle the wall of ego and residual anger that separates me from a deeper relationship with His ineffable nature and allow His healing presence to continue to fill in my *notwholeness*. Finally, there are prayers of gratitude for a God who is immanent and who constantly reveals Himself in surprising new ways—if only I stop and look and listen.

Thus, my spiritual journey continues. It has brought me from my head to my heart. Although I have not left my mind behind, in coming to my heart I have come to a lovely new country. And so much more is there yet to be discovered.

ELEVEN

Curative, Not Cured: Living With Prostate Cancer

HIKING THE CURATIVE TRAIL

I had finally completed all forty-two radiation treatments. It was certainly a relief to no longer have to make the daily 52-mile round trip between my home and the Radiation Oncology Center. But completing radiotherapy left a void. No more would I swoop into Rad Onc as a full-fledged member of an exclusive club, swipe my bar-coded ID at the reception desk, change into the hospital-issue pajama bottoms, and wait for Renato or Gretchen to arrive and summon me to the treatment table. I would miss the people and their light banter, which had helped distract me from the seriousness of what was happening.

The entire process had become a predictable and comforting liturgy. For a few minutes each weekday, I became the center of attention of a highly skilled and personable cadre of caregivers from whom no bodily secrets were hid. It was their expertise that ensured 6 million electron volts worth of energized photons were aimed at precisely the right spot "down there." Repeated five times per week over almost nine weeks, this rite could not help but create a bond between patient and therapist. Now that bond had been broken. Like a starry-eyed teenager, who has enjoyed a memorable few weeks at summer camp and grown close to his counselors, it was difficult for me to end this unusual but intense mountaintop experience without some sense of loss.

Undergoing radiotherapy had another valuable quality. It demonstrated tangibly that something significant was being accomplished: The cancer cells were being attacked aggressively with high-powered photons, and I was on the road to a cure. This sense of "doing something" helped maintain my morale. As it turned out, "doing something" was also meaningful to my family and friends. Now that it was over, many of them believed my Oncology Adventure Ride had been successful, rolling quietly onto the platform and coming to a stop. Radiotherapy was complete. It was time to get off. From their perspective, my cancer was now cured.

"Congratulations! You made it! You look great!" Over the next several weeks, variations on those enthusiastic exclamations were the happy refrain of many who greeted me. My immediate family was thrilled that it was all over, as they praised my courage and fortitude. At one level, of course, they were absolutely right. Something was indeed over. I had come through forty-two sessions of radiation with my body and facial appearance pretty much intact. Many people expressed surprise that I hadn't lost my hair. (Hair loss on the head, the universal symbol of cancer treatment, is the result of chemotherapy, not radiation.) No question about it: I was hungry to hear every affirmation of my health, and I deeply appreciated each expression of encouragement.

With radiotherapy complete, and its side effects hidden deep inside my body, I looked pretty much the same as I had before starting treatment. Whatever apprehension my supporters had felt during the past five months of diagnosis and treatment was now alleviated. I think many of them had transferred me from their "he's got cancer" category on their mental lists of worries and concerns over to their "he's cured!" box. This was not necessarily incorrect; the end of radiation was indeed a cause for celebration. Having seen me survive the Oncology Adventure Ride, many now bestowed on me the honorific title, "cancer survivor."

I may be a cancer survivor, but as I write this more than two years after completing radiotherapy, I still remain very much aboard the Oncology Adventure Ride. Treatment has not ended; it has merely taken on a more subtle form that is all but undetectable to others (except Susan, who knows my every facial expression and tic). In many ways this continuing journey has proven more challenging than radiotherapy.

For men like me, who have advanced prostate cancer, androgen deprivation therapy (ADT), known more euphemistically, if less accurately, as "hormone therapy," is a standard treatment that usually begins a month or two before radiation, and may continue for months or even years thereafter. The clinical goal of ADT is to shut off testosterone production in the testes, where 90 to 95 percent of the male hormone is produced. By the time my radiation course had ended, my testosterone level stood at 45 nanograms per milliliter (ng/ml); normal levels are anywhere between 250 and 850 ng/ml. With levels below 50 ng/ml considered "castrate," ADT was starting to do its job.

Three months after completing radiation and six months into hormone therapy, my PSA stood at less than 0.01 ng/mL, as close to zero as the test can reliably measure. At a follow-up exam, Dr. Massullo looked at the latest PSA lab results and exclaimed, "I'm ecstatic." While my clinical status at this point could hardly look better, the doctor was also thinking beyond the here and now. "Your testosterone level is still too high," he added, instantly neutralizing the enthusiasm of his earlier comment. "It should be in the teens. I'm going to give Dr. Hopkins a call and talk about adding in the anti-androgen."

I understood what was at the root of his concern. It all had to do with "curative intent." While "cured" means "restored to health," the definition of "curative" has a more ambiguous meaning, "tending toward healing," or as another definition puts it more bluntly, "never actually achieving a definitive cure." If "cured" were represented as a horizontal line on a piece of graph paper, "curative" would be drawn as a curve below that line, gradually coming tantalizingly close—but never actually touching—the "cured" boundary. The goal of "curative intent" in treating advanced prostate cancer is to eliminate all the cancer cells from the body, which is what radiation and ADT together are tasked to do. But there's no guarantee. It only takes a few maverick cells that have escaped the various forms of treatment to start the entire cancerous process over again, not necessarily in the prostate (which was pretty much fried by the radiation), but somewhere else in my body. Prostate cancer has amazing tenacity and when it recurs almost always migrates to bone.

In the end, curative intent is all about probabilities: doing whatever it takes to reduce the odds that the cancer will recur. The prostate cancer treatment community has defined metrics by which it identifies men with a high probability of prostate cancer recurrence: Stage T3 or T4 disease, Gleason score equal to 8 or greater, and/or PSA greater than 20. Both my stage (T4) and Gleason score (8) unfortunately qualified me as a member of this group. Given this reality, Dr. Massullo wanted to do everything possible to minimize the probability of any remaining cancer cells finding stray testosterone in my body on which to feast.

A phone call from Dr. Massullo a few days later confirmed that Dr. Hopkins and he indeed had seen eye-to-eye. Adding the anti-androgen drug to the ADT put me on a regimen called "combined androgen blockade" (CAB). The ADT drug does the primary work of shutting down testosterone production in the testes. The anti-androgen performs clean-up duty by preventing androgen receptors on cancer cells from binding to stray testosterone that may still be lingering in my body—especially the remaining 5 to 10 percent produced by the adrenal glands. Now on CAB, I felt a renewed awareness that "curative intent" was indeed different than "definitively cured." But it simply took too much energy to explain the subtle but crucial distinction between "cured" and "curative intent" to my family and friends, except of course, Susan, who was well aware of the difference. So, when someone said, "You're cured," I would just smile wanly.

While radiation is the overtly dramatic treatment, ADT and CAB are just as aggressive, especially in their side effects. But they are spread out over a much longer period, measured in months and years rather than weeks. Persistent hot flashes, the most noticeable side effect of living without testosterone, remind me every few hours that while I may be a cancer survivor, I am also still very much a cancer patient. Testosterone suppression will be a continuing part of my life for several years after radiation, and probably off and on thereafter for some years to come, until it stops working. At some point prostate cancer cells learn to thrive without testosterone—and some researchers believe some prostate cancer cells can even manufacture their own testosterone. This may happen in two years, ten years, or, hopefully, even longer. But for a person with high-grade cancer such as mine, recurrence is almost inevitable: At some point my cancer will become "castrate-resistant," which is the coldly clinical way of saying, "The cancer no longer requires your testosterone to grow. It's growing just fine all on its own. Therefore, the fact that you don't have testosterone is basically irrelevant." This possibility, if not eventuality, is the final reason why I cannot say, "I am cured," but only that I have been treated with "curative intent."

Once a man with advanced prostate cancer becomes castrate-resistant, more aggressive treatment strategies are required. This occasion also marks the gloomy passage from "curative intent," to the more ominous "palliative intent," the medical euphemism for "making the patient as comfortable as possible as the end draws near." However, the "end" may still be years away. There are pharmaceutical strategies such as ketoconazole and hydrocortisone that can put off the need to start actual chemotherapy for months and even years. And, as we've seen, there is an ever-growing variety of drugs such as Zytiga® and emerging immunotherapy such as Provenge® that can slow the cancer's progress as well. One of the oft-stated hopes of men with advanced prostate cancer—or any patient with cancer, for that matter—is that if they can forestall cancer's end game long enough, newer, more effective therapies still in development may become available. Participating in clinical trials is another possible way to slow the cancer's relentless march. Besides, in the meantime there are decent statistical odds that I may have died of something completely different, or have been run over by the proverbial truck.

> "Three quarters of men with prostate cancer will die of heart disease."
>
> —Mark Moyad, MD

One thing is certain: No therapy currently on the horizon will deliver a definitive cure. One hopeful sign, though, is the recent identification of "genotypes," sub-varieties, if you will, of prostate cancer. Understanding these different cancer strains at the genetic level may lead to "customized" treatment regimens based on the particular sub-type of cancer a man has. But as my friend Chuck keeps pointing out, cancer treatments are all about buying time. For me, that's what "curative intent" really means. It simply underscores the essential requirement to come to terms with one's own mortality. Once cancer became my partner, I was in the dance for keeps.

> The term "cancer free" does not mean that there are no cancer cells left in the body, only that existing technologies—in the case of prostate cancer, even the most sensitive PSA test—cannot detect them.

The benefits of buying time via testosterone suppression are substantial, but of course there are side effects to losing this important male hormone. Hiking the curative trail without testosterone in my body has substantial physical costs as the section "Complications of Androgen Deprivation Therapy" on page 193 illustrates. Until I began living without testosterone, I didn't realize just how much of our well-being and identity as men depends on it. Sexist claims are made by some men that women are ruled by their hormones. But really, testosterone rules men. I had been mentally prepared for the loss of ability to perform sexually, but it turns out that testosterone also drives libido. Without libido, the inability to perform sexually becomes irrelevant, because one doesn't even care about sex. Susan's gift to me through all this has been her immense compassion and loving patience with a husband, who has become—in the harshest of terms—a eunuch. We still love each other as much and as tenderly as ever, but now that my ability to express that love in the traditional physical manner is nonexistent, I regret the many opportunities for physical intimacy that I put off over the years because of distractions, petty disagreements, and disordered priorities.

Retrospectively, I see how my career, frequent travel, raising children, and commitments to outside activities (not to mention my frequent desire to vegetate in front of television) too often trumped sexual intimacy. But now it is probably too late. When ADT is administered even for a few months, its negative effect on a man's ability to experience erections is usually permanent—and the popular drugs for erectile dysfunction are often ineffective as well. Accordingly, Susan and I must find intimacy in other ways besides the obvious one. Happily, the human body has the capacity to express love in many ways.

A few years back, as I passed into my mid-50s, I often sympathized politely with my female contemporaries as they experienced menopause. But as a man, I had no real comprehension of the experience—until now. A term often used with only slightly disguised derision, "male menopause" or "manopause" (there's an official term, too: "andropause") now has a new, personal, and tangible reality. Every few hours my life is interrupted by a hot flash. Inexplicable mood swings are a new—and not terribly welcome—experience, and I often find myself welling up with tears during certain sentimental scenes in movies. My body has become increasingly feminized: I have lost much of my body hair, my genitals have shrunk, and my breasts have enlarged. In some small measure of compensation, though, Susan has told me how much softer my skin has become.

Nevertheless, I remain very much a male. I still need to shave (although I can go longer between shaves, if I desire), and my voice remains unchanged. And I've undertaken some efforts to compensate for the feminizing process. A few weeks following the completion of radiotherapy, I visited the barbershop. Seated in the chair, I suddenly and unaccountably blurted out, "a number two buzz cut, please." In just a few moments my gray and white hair lay on the shop's floor with only a few millimeters of fuzz remaining on my head. Looking in the mirror, it was suddenly 1969 again. I was back at the Navy base in Newport, Rhode Island, living through my first day at Officer Candidate School. My companions and I had watched appalled, as our long 1960s, Beatles-inspired locks were replaced by the regulation military-style haircut given to all new officer candidates. We had glanced warily at each other's newly shorn heads, almost too embarrassed to make eye contact. Forty years later, there was no embarrassment. That buzz cut somehow restored a bit of my diminished masculinity; I felt empowered and manly.

My short haircut helped me to regain some sense of masculinity, but it was not sufficient to express what had become my life-changing dance with advanced cancer. A few months following the buzz cut, my daughter-in-law Roxanne and I walked into Top Notch Tattoos in Elgin, Illinois. We had undertaken a mutual pact that we would each get a tattoo to mark major life events. Roxanne had completed her book on Alaska environmental history and had just sent it off to her publisher. I had completed radiotherapy. Following thirty minutes of mild discomfort, not dissimilar to the constant pricking of a blood draw, my tattoo was complete. Inscribed around my right wrist in light blue ink, the color representing prostate cancer, were the words "prostate cancer survivor" written in the flowing Elfish script invented by author JRR Tolkien for his *Lord of the Rings* trilogy. The inscription is intentionally inscrutable: not only so people will ask me about it, which they often do, but also to reflect the enigmatic nature of cancer itself.

Susan's loyal affection, the buzz cut, and the tattoo have helped ameliorate some of the physical and psychological losses created by my cancer and its treatment. But beyond the more obvious challenges of living with the aftereffects of radiation and ongoing androgen deprivation, there lurk other worrying possibilities.

COUNTERMEASURES: EXERCISE AND DIET

A testosterone-deprived body is subject to potentially more dangerous effects than hot flashes and loss of sexual capability. These include loss of muscle mass, along with loss of bone density that can lead to osteoporosis. Since I already had osteopinea, the precursor of osteoporosis, even before my cancer diagnosis, preventing the loss of still more bone mass during ADT was critical. This is why Dr. Hopkins had prescribed quarterly infusions of Zometa®, (often administered as Reclast® to post-menopausal women). Other side effects of testosterone suppression, including weight gain and the heightened possibility of diabetes and heart problems, were equally concerning. To me, the most sobering of all were the ominous words of a paper published in late 2007, which stated cryptically, "Greater baseline BMI is independently associated with higher PCSM in men with locally advanced prostate cancer." Translated: If you have advanced prostate cancer, and a high Body Mass Index (mine was moderately high—about

31), you are more likely to die from prostate cancer (PCSM, prostate cancer-specific mortality) than men who weigh less. And this was even before ADT could begin to work its wonders by encouraging additional weight gain. Clearly, I needed to think about aggressive countermeasures.

Complications of Androgen Deprivation Therapy

Men often experience fatigue, loss of energy and emotional distress from androgen suppression treatment. Hormonal therapy may significantly impair quality of life, particularly in men who had no symptoms beforehand and whose cancer has not metastasized. Common side effects of androgen suppression drugs include:

- Hot flashes, which may go away over time
- Osteoporosis, the loss of bone density. A number of medications, especially bisphosphonates, are available to help prevent or reduce bone loss
- Decrease in HDL ("good" cholesterol) levels
- Loss of muscle mass
- Weight gain
- Decreased mental alertness
- Fatigue and depression
- Swelling and tenderness of the breasts (gynecomastia)
- Anemia (low red blood cell count)
- Sexual dysfunction and loss of sex drive

In addition, there is growing evidence that androgen deprivation therapy increases risk for heart attack, stroke, and diabetes.

Source: New York Times Health Guides

The cancer may have stripped away my illusion of being able to control every situation, but that didn't mean I lacked power over important aspects of my life. Perhaps one of the reasons we like to imagine that we control our destinies is that we are too often incapable of controlling the small habits of our everyday lives. There is a host of conscious decisions we can make if we can summon the requisite will and self-discipline. This is easy to say, but more difficult to implement. I have focused on two self-disciplines that probably every sentient adult male should be paying attention to, regardless of whether he has cancer: diet and exercise. Now, with hormone therapy threatening to add weight as it simultaneously diminished muscle mass and bone density, I was truly motivated to move (in all the definitions of the word) beyond good intentions.

Exercise was the easier variable to address because it was already a habit. As a younger man, I had started each day with running, and my business travels had taken me to many interesting jogging venues around the world. Between the late 1980s and mid 1990s in-line skating was easier on my joints than running—but not on my shins, kneecaps, and two of my front teeth. Age and common sense eventually put an end to the skating, and since then I have worked out at the gym four to five days a week. Treadmills, rowing machines, and weights are my partners, if not exactly my friends.

Along with the journal articles that warned of the negative correlation between obesity and advanced prostate cancer, there were other, more encouraging studies describing the benefits of exercise for men living a testosterone-deprived life. One such article stated,

> *These results support that exercise has beneficial effects on muscle strength, aerobic fitness and QOL [quality of life] for patients with PC [prostate cancer] receiving ADT or radiation therapy as exercise may counter some of the morbid side effects of these treatments.*

Another paper focused on what was the best kind of exercise for me:

> *Resistance exercise reduces fatigue and improves quality of life and muscular fitness in men with prostate cancer receiving androgen deprivation therapy.*

A study conducted by the Harvard School of Public Health and University of California, San Francisco, concluded that for all prostate cancer patients, "Men who did more vigorous activity had the lowest risk of dying from the disease."

With potential bone and muscle mass loss looming, it was definitely time to up my game at the gym. I met with Adam, a personal trainer, the week after starting radiotherapy. After explaining prostate cancer to this virile 29 year old, who had only a foggy notion of what a prostate was, much less having encountered anyone with a cancerous one, I said, "Now, unlike all your other clients, I'm likely to lose strength rather than gain it while we're working out the next few weeks."

"Say, what?"

"Yeah," I explained, "I'm undergoing radiation and hormone therapy for the cancer. Both of these create fatigue, and I may get weaker as time progresses. Don't get me wrong. I'm going to work hard. I just wanted to make sure you knew that I may not respond like your typical 62-year-old client, much less your typical 30- or 40-year-old client."

"That's OK; no one's ever told me about this stuff before, but I'll make sure to keep your abilities and strength in mind as we proceed," he responded. "Let's get to work."

Work we did: an hour twice a week over four weeks. I performed the same sequence of exercises by myself on the days we weren't training together. Adam focused on my abdominal core: stretching and dynamic balance, mostly using an exercise ball and a few weights. Even though none of these exercises was particularly vigorous, keeping my muscles in dynamic equilibrium was a physical challenge, more tiring than my traditional workouts on the weight machines. Spurred on by visions of desiccated muscles and hollowed-out bone, I continue to persist three to five times a week at the gym. Are my muscles stronger, my bones as dense as before? There's only the evidence that, even as the ADT continues, I can work out longer and harder than ever. That's been enormously positive for my morale. I feel like there's at least a small part of my life that I have been able to snatch back from the cancer and the drugs. It helps make the dance with this ugly disease more balanced—and perhaps a bit more graceful.

Changing my diet has been more challenging. I still have no idea if my dietary habits over the years were among the proximate causes of my cancer, although they were probably a contributing factor. I had long known that being thirty pounds overweight and consuming red meat and saturated fats of every variety were not great lifestyle choices. Unfortunately, theoretical knowledge rarely provides sufficient motivation to change.

Having long given lip service to the idea of altering my diet and losing weight, the cancer added more than conceptual urgency. The nutritionist at the Radiation Oncology Center had said that I should avoid losing weight while undergoing radiotherapy, and I had happily complied with her recommendation. But that excuse had now ended; it was time to get serious about at least maintaining, if not losing, weight in the face of my body's now amplified ability to add on pounds. If avoiding weight gain was the first dietary issue, the second was equally important: I didn't want to consume anything that could accelerate my cancer's return.

Notwithstanding an enormous multi-billion dollar industry of diet systems, books, videos, machines, nostrums, gurus, supplements, and drugs, my engineer's mind had reduced the weight loss equation to a single sentence: "Eat fewer calories while eating healthier foods." Every meal every day should be a sequence of conscious nutritional decisions. I wanted to be aware of the caloric impact of each choice—not just on my weight, but also on how the better nutrition might buy me more time. The idea of eating better to live longer has become more effective than simply losing weight to motivate me to make healthy choices.

Searching the terms "diet and prostate cancer" in the professional literature disclosed numerous papers on their relationship, but definitive conclusions, much less any agreement among authors, were harder to find. Judging by the large number of published articles, researchers are indeed busy studying how various foods influence the causes, prevention, and course of prostate cancer. But clear linkages between what we eat and the disease itself continue to be elusive. The enormous variety of foods that comprise the modern American diet makes it effectively impossible to demonstrate a direct connection between a particular food—or even a component of food—and prostate cancer. In one paper with the thought-provoking title, "Diet After Diagnosis and the Risk of Prostate Cancer Progression, Recurrence, and Death (United States)," the authors cautiously, if somewhat obviously, note that, yes indeed, diet may affect the cancer's eventual course. As if searching for something more useful to say, the authors endorsed fish and tomato sauce as "offering some protection [against further progression of the cancer]."

Another article included a helpful list of what's "protective" and what's "risky" in terms of contracting prostate cancer in the first place. The authors observe,

> *There are several potential protective dietary factors for prostate cancer incidence, including tomatoes, cruciferous vegetables, carotenoids, vitamin E, selenium, fish, long-chain marine omega-3 fatty acids, soy, and polyphenols; whereas milk, dairy, calcium, zinc at high doses, saturated fat, and red or grilled meats may increase risk.*

After hearing my doctors stress the importance of calcium to offset the bone-weakening effects of ADT, it was discouraging to see that dairy and calcium "may increase risk [of prostate cancer]." This conundrum usefully demonstrates why the search for a dietary silver bullet with respect to prostate cancer (as well as other cancers) is so complicated: What's good for the preventive goose may not apply to the post-diagnosis gander. The authors acknowledge the calcium problem, happily coming down on the side of common sense, stating:

> *Men receiving hormone therapy for prostate cancer are at greater risk of osteoporosis and are often recommended to consume bisphosphonates and calcium supplements. This recommendation remains appropriate given that (1) researchers estimate that 10% to 40% of men with advanced prostate cancer have osteoporotic fractures depending upon duration of hormone therapy; and (2) no data exist specifically addressing whether calcium consumption after prostate cancer diagnosis affects further risk of progression.*

The phrase "no data exist" underscores the complexity of validating a clear relationship between what we eat and the probable course of a cancer. This reality is also a cautionary tale for the frequent infomercial and email claims that this particular food or that particular supplement is the secret to preventing or even curing prostate cancer. The virtues of açaí berries, green tea, pomegranate juice, extract of saw palmetto leaf, among others, continue to be extolled. In the memorable words of Dr. Hopkins when I asked him about the value of pomegranate juice in reducing the odds of my cancer's recurrence, he replied, "Well, it can't hurt."

So, if there are no obvious dietary solutions, where does this leave those of us with advanced prostate cancer? The answer is simple: dietary common sense. Or, as the authors quoted earlier state more formally,

> *It would be prudent to emphasize a diet consisting of a wide variety of plant-based foods and fish; this is similar to what is recommended (and what is better established) for the primary prevention of heart disease. More succinctly: what's good for the heart is good for the prostate.*

Sticking to plant-based foods and fish for simultaneous heart and prostate health is excellent advice, although it's challenging to translate into consistent daily practice. Since I am not an organized, calorie-counting guy, I try to follow some simple practices:

1. Avoid processed foods as much as possible. Stick to what is generally stocked at the side and back walls of most grocery stores.
2. Steer clear of "white" ingredients—especially flour and sugar—as much as possible, since white usually means highly processed.
3. Eat lots of green and brightly colored vegetables, beans of all kinds, and acquire a taste for tofu.

This list is not a prescription; it's more a reflection of consciously engaging with my diet instead of my years-long habit of thoughtlessly eating whatever struck my fancy.

I encounter bumps in the road and occasional detours in my quest to ingrain healthy dietary habits. I miss the many staples of the American diet on which I feasted for so many years, especially hamburgers, steak, dry salami, brats, and San Francisco sourdough bread. Occasionally, that love is briefly rekindled, especially with cake and ice cream.

INTO UNEXPLORED TERRITORY

It is beyond cliché: There is far more to health (and to disease) than just its physical qualities. I have already described cancer's impact on my personal relationships and on my spiritual outlook on life. Prostate cancer and its treatment have had a profound psychological impact as well. My disease has affected my mental state, my thoughts and behaviors—and my self-image. This is not just about mental attitude. ADT drugs can negatively affect mental sharpness in some men. Clinical depression among men with advanced prostate cancer—either on or off ADT—is unfortunately all too common.

Even though cancer is my constant companion, I must still live in the everyday world. As a technology marketing consultant, my livelihood depends on maintaining topnotch mental acuity and creative thinking skills. My hobby of landscape photography depends on my ability to see what others may miss, and compose images of interest and originality. How might the cancer, and even more worryingly, the androgen deprivation, affect those skills and abilities? To explore these questions, I turned again to the medical research literature.

As I noted earlier, thousands of journal articles dealing with every conceivable clinical and technological aspect of prostate cancer are published each year. This is good. The more people there are working on the problem, the sooner more effective treatments will be developed. Given prostate cancer's mental and emotional impact on men's self-image, I was sure I'd find a large body of journal literature discussing the psychological impact of prostate cancer. The truth is that not much work has been done on this subject, although some researchers are aware of this problem. In 2007, a group of psychiatrists and oncologists published a meta-analysis of psychological research performed between 1994 and 2006. The authors note the imbalance between clinical and psychological research, articulating what I felt after my mostly fruitless journal search:

> *Puzzlingly, almost all research has been devoted to physical aspects and side effects of treatment and very little to such psychological features as emotional distress, coping and psychiatric morbidity. Psychological adjustment is complex, given the disease's potential trajectory — from the point of diagnosis, with its immediate impact, to the phase of palliative care, with its attendant existential issues.*

Ah, yes, the "attendant existential issues" such as loss of sexual capability, loss of male self image, loss of mental sharpness, and increased depression and anxiety. The authors conclude,

> *We found few studies of substance among the 60 we examined to draw conclusions about psychological adjustment to prostate cancer and its treatment. This is in marked contrast to the picture in breast cancer. While some patterns have emerged, many gaps remain to be filled.*

The comparison to women's health issues—particularly breast cancer—was striking. It reminded me just how far the medical, research, and therapeutic communities addressing men's health issues have yet to traverse. Doctors and medical technologists are far more comfortable operating on the solid ground of their clinical expertise than on the comparatively marshy land of the psychosocial and sexual issues created by this disease. As a result, the topic tends to be addressed only perfunctorily among doctor, patient, and the patient's spouse. So like most men before me, I was left to strike out on my own into this mostly unexplored territory.

Finding a clear map of the psycho-sociology of prostate cancer is even more challenging when it comes to separating out discussions about the emotional effects of androgen deprivation therapy. One paper's data that consisted of "quality of life" questionnaires filled out by 178 men with advanced prostate cancer, half of whom were on ADT and half of whom were not, came to an unsurprising (and to one who is actually experiencing ADT, basically trivial) conclusion:

> *Androgen deprivation therapy for asymptomatic men with locally advanced prostate cancer or PSA relapse after local therapy produced worse quality of life outcomes compared to no hormone therapy.*

The authors go on to note that combined androgen blockade (CAB) may have even more negative consequences than androgen deprivation alone:

> *Fatigue, emotional distress, decreased physical functioning and impaired overall quality of life [that] were most pronounced in patients receiving combined androgen blockade...*

This dry, scientific language keeps the emotional impact of these conclusions at bay: good for researchers, less so for men like me, who are actually experiencing the dramatic effects of testosterone suppression. While this paper explained the scientific basis of ADT's effects, it offered no practical guidance as to how men might deal more effectively with androgen deprivation's psychological impact. Are there other strategies for coping with body feminization beyond getting a buzz cut and a tattoo? What approaches might be useful in dealing with the loss of not only sexual ability, but also of sexual interest? What about the significant impact of loss of sexuality on the patient's partner? Are there techniques that might help prevent or at least minimize the loss of mental sharpness caused by ADT?

One article, based on detailed interviews of fifteen Israeli men undergoing ADT, suggested that these authors truly understood the profound psychological consequences of testosterone suppression:

> *Despite the growing body of research on the psychosocial problems generated by prostate cancer, as yet no comprehensive understanding exists of the tactics that patients adopt for coping with them.... An understanding of such coping strategies is particularly warranted in the case of advanced prostate cancer patients receiving hormonal therapy because of the unique nature and special severity of the psychosocial problems that they face.*

This sobering paper described how men on ADT had developed basic coping mechanisms—disguising, diverting, and avoiding—in the three major areas of their lives affected by ADT:

1. A feminized body
2. Extinguished sexuality
3. New constraints on intimate relations with their spouses

There they were: the same "big three" changes that had occurred in my own life. At least the researchers had acknowledged them as significant psychological stressors.

Another group of authors, one of whom has advanced prostate cancer and has experienced androgen deprivation therapy, writes, "Patients on ADT despair because they no longer feel or function fully as men." But there is a further burden to experiencing ADT: the perceived social stigma of chemical castration. These authors go on to observe that are few positive qualities to being a eunuch in our society:

> *Inaccurate, antiquated, and negative stereotypes of castrated men—implicitly illustrated by the misuse of the term "eunuch" to indicate a completely powerless person—are perpetuated because of society's general ignorance of contemporary castrations. The language of emasculation remains pejorative and shameful.*

They argue that language is a powerful force, and that society at large, and especially the press, should work to change society's attitude toward emasculation in terms of attitudes and public awareness:

> *We surmise that they [men on ADT] are driven underground largely because of a stigmatization perpetrated by the metaphorical language used by those unaware of their existence. The invisibility of the medically emasculated leads to further ignorance on the part of the public, causing the use of this offensive language to go unchecked, and driving castrated individuals deeper into hiding.... It is necessary that we reclaim the language of emasculation for the individuals to whom it refers, so that men diagnosed with prostate cancer can consider treatment options free from the fear of stigma, and so that those men already androgen-deprived do not feel the need to hide.*

Equally significant is how both prostate cancer and androgen deprivation in particular affect the spousal relationship:

> *ADT both emasculates and feminizes. Men can disguise most of the anatomic alterations caused by ADT with a carefully chosen wardrobe. They cannot, however, hide ADT's effects in one place that is an integral part of many men's lives—the bedroom.*

Prostate cancer, like breast cancer, is a "relationship disease" because it directly affects persons beyond the patient himself. Where ADT is concerned, the too often forgotten party is the spouse or significant other of the man being treated. Obviously I have lost my sexual capabilities and interest, but Susan has lost as much, perhaps more. In my experience, this significant physical and psychological loss and its impact on one's spouse is rarely, if ever, discussed directly in any of the literature given to men prior to their decision to undergo ADT. Basically, it's left up to the man and his partner to figure out the sexual and relational consequences of ADT for themselves—and, too often, only after hormone therapy has already taken effect. One study notes, "There is growing evidence that the diagnosis of prostate cancer has important adverse psychosocial effects on both the patient and his partner." It concludes:

> *Partners of cancer patients experience significant psychological distress, perhaps suffering as many adjustment problems as the patients themselves. A cross-sectional study of [prostate cancer] patients and their spouses found that spouses reported significantly greater psychological distress than the patients themselves.*

Psychological, social, relational: These are the stressors that accompany the physical reality of prostate cancer, not to mention the additional stresses of androgen deprivation therapy. A big question (and one that is implied but not addressed in most of these papers) remains: Are these well-documented physical, psychological, and relational downsides of testosterone suppression worth its curative intent?

I don't think this question will ever be answered definitively in a scientific or therapeutic setting, no matter what data ultimately get collected. Testosterone suppression therapy halts the growth of androgen-dependent cancer cells for some period that can range from months to years. It definitely satisfies my friend Chuck's criterion that the point of any cancer therapy is to buy time. In my own case, ADT combined with radiation means I have a 93 percent statistical probability of still being alive in five years, although the odds decline after that. But this therapy also leads to all the physical and psychological downsides just discussed.

In the end, it's a question that can be answered only by the man with the cancer, ideally with the full participation of his partner, if he has one. This is a place where general principles or rules become irrelevant. Only the man with prostate cancer, who is facing androgen deprivation, and his significant other know— or at least can posit—all the physical and emotional variables involved. The authors of the Israeli study describe the tradeoff that is the most powerful coping mechanism of all:

> *The most commonly used cognitive coping tactic, and the one to which the interviewees attributed the greatest efficacy, was convincing themselves that the physical changes were a worthy sacrifice for staying alive.*

It's really a simple economy: Additional time is purchased at the price of diminished manhood. As for myself: So be it. Coping, like diet and exercise, has its upsides. Life is laced with uncertainty and ambiguity for every person, cancer patient or not. I successfully held that reality at arm's length for too many years. But I am starkly reminded of life's twists, turns, and uncertainties—and the often unpleasant tradeoffs each of us must make—each time I look in the mirror at my changed body, or see a TV commercial for erectile dysfunction remedies … or, far, far better, when Susan and I embrace, both in loving awareness that the additional time we can remain close together is the most precious gift of all.

A LIFE ANNEALED

Annealing is "a heat treatment wherein a material is altered, causing changes in its properties such as strength and hardness." It's an ancient process of heating glass or various metals and then cooling them slowly in order to toughen them and reduce their brittleness. "Annealing" has come often to mind as I have reflected and written on the impact of all that has occurred since hearing those scary words in January 2009. First, there was "prostate cancer," then "Gleason 8 aggressive cancer," then "anti-androgen," then "advanced cancer," then "radiotherapy," then "androgen deprivation therapy," then "combined androgen blockade." Each phase of the Oncology Adventure Ride has added more heat. Now with radiotherapy a memory, and doctor visits reduced in frequency, and continuing to live each day without testosterone, I am metaphorically in the cooling phase: learning to live on a day-to-day basis with the reality of diminished manhood, and always aware that at any time the cancer may return—what some have called the "overhang." But I am also living with the full appreciation of what it means to dance with cancer. I am living with a new understanding of how critically important and vital relationships are—especially with my wife, who has been just as affected by my cancer as I have.

The objective of annealing is to reduce stress and, in the case of metals, to make them easier to mold and bend. The metaphor holds. By eliminating my misapprehension that I was an independent, self-sustaining person fully in charge of my destiny, cancer has left me physically, spiritually, and psychologically vulnerable—and malleable. And that is all right: Vulnerability has increased my willingness to accept—and to live with—my weaknesses and my limitations. Even better, it has made me more open to the love and affection of those who surround me—and of God, who is indeed nearby.

None of us knows how our lives will ultimately unfold—even though I once believed I knew. I now know only that it will play out one day at a time. In the presence of a disease, yes; but also in the presence of God, of a community, of friends, of family, and of a loving wife. I am thankful for this, for this is indeed sufficient.

EPILOGUE

The Future of Prostate Cancer

We baby boomers have been the demographic force behind substantial changes in American culture since we began appearing on the scene in 1946. In the 1950s, young boomers influenced early television programming and advertising as our parents moved to growing suburbs and became post-war consumers. Coming of age in the 1960s, we shaped popular music, print and electronic media, and impacted long-established attitudes toward authority, so much so that "baby boomers" were designated *Time* magazine's Man of the Year in 1967. Draft-age boomers comprised the engine of Vietnam protests and effectively drove Lyndon Johnson from office. By the mid-1970s, as Vietnam faded from public consciousness, we embraced a new environmental awareness and confidence in our generation's ability to change the world—ostensibly for the better. By the 1980s, the visionaries of the 1960s and 1970s had morphed into full-fledged consuming adults and began forming families. Andrew Sullivan has argued that this was the moment when boomers divided into opposing political camps, resulting in the "culture wars" and bitter partisanship that defines political dialog today.

But as we boomers move into our seventh decade, the issue becomes less how our generation will turn culture on its head and more about how we will deal with aging, disease, and death. One thing is certain: Even though policymakers fret about how the sheer size of the boomer cohort are likely to bankrupt Social Security and Medicare, we will continue to celebrate our eternal youth. We are the generation for whom Bob Dylan's song, "Forever Young," remains an anthem. Our collective attitude of eternal youthfulness motivated the American Association of Retired Persons to become an acronym, AARP, since many of us see the very word "retired" as anathema, applicable only to our parents and grandparents.

Behind this cultural façade, however, the reality is that we boomers are aging at exactly the same rate as our forebears. How are we, who have always seemed to be able to bend American culture to our collective will, going to deal with the inevitability of physical decline?

Boomers are infamous for their efforts to stave off the aging process. We have long placed a premium on health and fitness: from the jogging boom of the 1980s to the 24-hour gyms common today, to say nothing of our role as active participants in the $35 billion per year weight loss industry. Of course, many aging boomers in good health will simply choose to deny the consequences of growing old. It's still too early to tell, but if "50 was the new 40" for boomers, there's little reason to doubt that "60 will be the new 50." (And for us leading-edge boomers, "70 will be the new 60.") We are likely to attack the problem of aging with the same self-centered gusto we've approached politics, culture, and consumerism. A 2004 study on boomer attitudes about health issues underscores our active engagement when it comes to our well-being:

> *Boomers will not quietly accept either health problems or problems in getting healthcare. Demand for more resources to meet their healthcare needs and new research into the health problems afflicting them will increase. Although development of some health conditions may be an inevitable part of aging, it is unlikely that Boomers will passively accept this fact.*

But regardless of attitude, boomers cannot transcend the harsh reality that everything, including our generation, eventually runs its course and dies. The reality of aging will eventually trump even the most hardened cases of denial. My cancer is merely a harbinger of what will happen to increasing numbers of boomers as our cohort ages. As noted earlier, the 2009 study examining the implications of an aging population on cancer diagnoses states, "The number of cancer cases, particularly in older and minority individuals, is expected to vastly increase over the next two decades." Even with ongoing and often significant therapeutic breakthroughs, the authors project an annual growth of prostate cancer, reaching more than 380,000 cases by 2030, when the lagging edge of boomers born in 1964 turns 66.

"Between 2010 and 2030, a 67% increase in cancer incidence is anticipated for patients age 65 years or older (1.0 million to 1.6 million instances), compared with only an 11% increase in cancer incidence anticipated for patients younger than the age of 65 years (0.63 million to 0.67 million instances)."

— Benjamin D. Smith

What do our ingrained attitudes about eternal youth and health portend for those of us diagnosed with prostate cancer, or any kind of cancer, for that matter? How will a person, who has been able to control almost everything about his or her personal life, react upon hearing the four scary words, "You have [this kind of] cancer"? Will he or she respond as I did? Initially I felt confusion and fear, but ultimately I had to acknowledge the life-changing reality of my disease, and along with it, my mortality. Will this stark news lead to big questions like "Why is life unfair?" Or will some of our generation simply party on, hedonistically deciding "Tomorrow or sometime after that we may die of cancer, but let's continue to have a good time right now"? Cancer's innate ability to create dread suggests this latter scenario is unlikely.

Aligning themselves with the assumptions noted above, a group of researchers looked into the issue of prostate cancer in this generation, noting in their introduction that boomers are *better educated, have higher incomes, and are wealthier than their predecessors.... [They] are thought to place a high value on quality of life, and have a higher propensity to consume healthcare services than previous generations.... Media portrayals stereotype Baby Boomers as health-conscious and placing a high value on quality of life.*

The researchers go on to explain that they want to understand "how this generation may or may not be changing the face of prostate cancer and its treatment." They acknowledge that the "study has some limitations, [because] the baby boomer generation is just entering the age when prostate cancer is diagnosed, and thus our analysis represents the early experience of this generation." The assumption that boomers will alter the face of prostate cancer treatment as they have other things fails to be borne out so far. When it comes to choosing among cancer treatments, boomers are behaving as conventionally as their fathers:

Other investigations into the characteristics of the Baby Boomer cohort demonstrate that reality is more complex than the stereotypes of this generation would suggest.... Our study suggests that, in contrast to media stereotypes, Baby Boomers diagnosed with prostate cancer do not choose different treatments from men born earlier who were diagnosed at the same age.

So, at least for the boomers diagnosed thus far, when it comes to actually facing the life altering realities of prostate cancer (and other cancers), the evidence suggests that clinical realities will trump generational personality—even for this most ideological of generations.

While medical pragmatism may drive treatment choices even for boomers, there is little reason to expect that this generation will remain quiet on other important issues related to cancer—especially research and in keeping with our demographic character, passionate advocacy. Philanthropist Michael Milken is certainly one of the generation's leaders of prostate cancer research and advocacy. In 1993, Milken was diagnosed with aggressive, advanced prostate cancer at the unusually early age of 43. When diagnosed, the cancer had already spread to his lymph nodes, and he was given a grim prognosis of less than two years to live. Following a prostatectomy, he underwent radiation and androgen deprivation. As of this writing in 2012, he is still very much alive. He founded the Prostate Cancer Foundation, which has become an exemplar among disease-specific foundations, awarding "out of the box" grants to scientists with creative but unconventional ideas for research unlikely to be funded by traditional, government sources. Applying a boomer's "let's not just accept the status quo" mentality, Milken's money and efforts, in the words of a 2004 *Fortune* magazine article,

> *"Changed the culture of [medical] research," says Andrew von Eschenbach, director of the National Cancer Institute. "He created a sense of urgency that focused on results and shortened the timeline. It took a business mindset to shake things up. What he's done is now the model."*

Of course, few boomers have a net worth exceeding $2 billion available to fund creative research efforts. But for a generation that has identified and attacked entrenched political, environmental, and social norms, the cultural attitude toward cancer—and prostate cancer, in particular—are obvious targets for transformation. It's safe to forecast that in the coming years, as thousands of boomers are diagnosed, they, their significant others, and their families will collectively drive changes in research and funding priorities, even as they simultaneously increase public awareness of the disease.

In the research already underway, perhaps the most important change might be in how prostate cancer is screened and detected. Because the existence of a prostate tumor can be detected earlier via the PSA test, the test has become an important component in reducing prostate cancer mortality rates. But as the recent controversial recommendation of the United States Preventive Services Task Force to discontinue PSA screening illustrates, the test is far from being a diagnostic silver bullet. PSA levels are affected by conditions other than cancer, including prostatitis and BPH, urinary tract infections, and even how recently a man has had sex. More critically, PSA cannot discriminate between indolent, slow-growing cancers and more aggressive tumors. This latter shortcoming has led to overtreatment, including the unnecessary removal of slow-growing cancers confined to the prostate. Finally, there's the problem that I share with about 3 percent of men diagnosed with prostate cancer: aggressive cancer that occurs with no detectable change in PSA levels.

The ambiguity of PSA testing was demonstrated in early 2009 by the simultaneous release of two studies about the relationship of PSA screening to prostate cancer mortality. One study, conducted in the US, concluded that PSA testing had not decreased prostate cancer mortality rates at all. The second study, conducted in Europe, concluded the opposite, although the decrease in mortality was small. Since then, urologists have been counseling confused men that they should simply ignore the ambiguity and continue to get regular PSA tests if they're over 50, have a family history, or are African American. One upshot of the studies is clear: The medical community and the men it serves need a definitive test to detect the presence of prostate cancer, as well one that can discriminate between indolent and aggressive forms of the disease.

Happily, there has been some progress on this front. Genetic biomarkers found in urine have emerged as a promising method for detection and discrimination among various forms of prostate cancer. Researchers have recently located key biomarkers that "outperformed serum PSA or PCA3 [thus far] favored alone in detecting prostate cancer." While a standard urine test to detect prostate cancer has not yet arrived at the local urologist's office, it's clear that more accurate tests that supplement or even replace the PSA test may become available soon enough to help large numbers of aging male boomers.

Because there are at least twenty-seven distinct sub-varieties ("genotypes") of prostate cancer, there is the hope that treatment programs will be developed that are optimized to the characteristics of a particular sub-type. Diagnosis based on genotype could also reduce the confusion over which treatment to administer when, which, as noted in Chapter 8, will become increasingly important as new pharmaceuticals are developed. Diagnostic tools that are further into the future may include implantable nanotechnology, a monitoring system that could chart "the course of the tumor growth and spread, how it is responding to treatment, whether it has metastasized or is ready to do so." For those of us worrying about the tradeoff between ADT side effects and cancer progression, a technology such as this would be invaluable both medically and psychologically.

Finally, it is in our generation's area of specialization—transforming cultural values—where we boomers arguably can have our greatest impact. As increasing numbers of boomers are diagnosed, it's safe to predict that prostate cancer will eventually emerge from behind the shadow of breast cancer awareness. Lifting of societal taboos about breast cancer began back in 1974 when Betty Ford and Happy Rockefeller (both assuredly not boomers) went public with their breast cancers and mastectomies, urging women to receive regular examinations. Although widespread awareness of prostate cancer and its consequences lags by several years, it's a safe prediction that boomers will advance awareness. Until the early 1990s, the word "prostate" was simply not uttered in polite company. Lately, well-known men such as Rudy Guiliani and John Kerry announced to the world when they were diagnosed with prostate cancer and how they were treated, advising men over 50 to take a PSA test. Other boomers have become fully engaged in the cause, such as tennis star John MacInroe, whose father had prostate cancer. Dana Jennings, an editor at the *New York Times*, performed an invaluable service for numerous men when he blogged regularly in 2008 and 2009 about his diagnosis and treatment for aggressive prostate cancer. Dennis Hopper, the star of 1969's *Easy Rider*, died of advanced prostate cancer in 2010—a wake-up call to many who had equated Hopper with their youthful fancy.

Our frequently strident and always active generation surely will see to it that that funding for research, public education, and screening increases as prostate cancer begins to affect an ever-larger number of men. The boomers who marched for political causes in the 1960s now walk designated courses in various cities to raise funds for a variety of cancer-related causes, most significantly the 3-day Avon Breast Cancer Walk. Various prostate cancer walks and runs are now cropping up as more men participate actively in the cause. These are hopeful beginnings, as men gain courage to tell other men about the consequences of ignoring what's going on "down there."

In the not too distant future, the trajectory of prostate cancer diagnosis, treatment, research, awareness, and, ultimately, its cure will surely bend to the collective will and concerted actions of this engaged generation that so greatly values its health and longevity.

But what of my own future? This is the question that each man with prostate cancer, and especially those of us with advanced disease, must ask. From here on out, for the rest of my life, no day will go by when I am not conscious of my cancer, which although quiescent as I write these words, will always lurk within me. What do I do with this unrelenting threat of its return? Will it be next month? A year from now? Five or ten years from now? Any attempt to predict is foolhardy. Any doctor who claims to know how much time any man with this disease has remaining is arrogantly mistaken.

So, cancer keeps me firmly rooted in the present: today. The saying is a cliché because it is true: Today is a gift. The tools and treatments available to me right now are providing many more todays than if I had been diagnosed just ten or fifteen years ago. And those diagnosed after me will enjoy an even greater number of todays because of the steady progress being made on so many fronts against this insidious disease.

And by consciously savoring each of these todays—one at a time—I can go to sleep each night in peace, knowing that regardless of what happens in the future, today was sufficient reward. Tomorrow will take care of itself.

Bibliography

CHAPTER ONE

National Cancer Institute website, 2011. Available at www. cancer.gov. Accessed October 2011.

Patterson, James. *The Dread Disease: Cancer in Modern American Culture.* Cambridge: Harvard University Press, 1987.

CHAPTER TWO

Barry, Michael J. "Screening for Prostate Cancer—The Controversy that Refuses to Die." *New England Journal of Medicine* 360 (March 2009): 1351–54.

Bud, R.F. "Strategy in American Cancer Research After World War II: A Case Study." *Social Studies of Science* 8 (1978): 425.

Chan, June, Meir Stamfer, and Edward Giovannucci. "What Causes Prostate Cancer? A Brief Summary of the Epidemiology." *Seminars in Cancer Biology* 8 (1998): 263–73.

Chu, T. Ming. "Prostate Specific Antigen (PSA): The Historical Perspective." *McGill Journal of Medicine* 2 (1996): 122–26.

De Marzo, A.M., E.A. Platz, S. Sutcliffe, and others. "Inflammation in Prostate Carcinogenesis." *Nature Reviews Cancer* 7 (April 2007): 256–69.

Denmeade, Samuel R., and John T. Isaacs. "A History of Prostate Cancer Treatment." *Nature Reviews Cancer* 2 (2002): 394.

Klein, Eric A., and Robert Silverman. "Inflammation, Infection, and Prostate Cancer." *Current Opinion in Urology* 18 (2008): 315–19.

Limonta, P. "The Biology of Gonadotropin Hormone-Releasing Hormone: Role in the Control of Tumor Growth and Progression in Humans." *Frontiers of Neuroendocrinology* 24 (December 2003): 279–95.

Lytton, Bernard. "Prostate Cancer: A Brief History and the Discovery of Hormonal Ablation Treatment." *The Journal of Urology* (June 2001): 1859.

McDavid, Kathleen. "Prostate Cancer Incidence and Mortality Rates and Trends in the United States and Canada." *Public Health Reports* 119 (March–April 2004): 117.

Roberts, R.O., E.J. Bergstralh, S.E. Bass, and others. "Prostatitis as a Risk Factor for Prostate Cancer." *Epidemiology* A5 (January 2004): 93–8.

The New York Times (New York) 11 January 2009.

CHAPTER THREE

The New Prostate Cancer InfoLink Social Network website, 2011. Available at www.prostatecancerinfolink.net. Accessed October 2011.

CHAPTER FOUR

Cooperberg, M.R., D.J. Pasta, E.P. Elkin, and others. "The University of California, San Francisco, Cancer of the Prostate Risk Assessment Score: A Straightforward and Reliable Predictor of Disease Recurrence After Radical Prostatectomy." *Journal of Urology* 173 (2005): 1938–42.

Homberg, L., A. Bill-Axelson, and others. "A Randomized Trial Comparing Radical Prostatectomy with Watchful Waiting in

Early Prostate Cancer." *New England Journal of Medicine* 347 (2002): 781–89.

Khan, Masood A., and Alan W. Partin. "Expectant Management of Prostate Cancer." *Reviews in Urology* 5 (Fall 2003): 247–50.

Thompson, I.M., D.K. Pauler, P.J. Goodman, and others. "Prevalence of Prostate Cancer Among Men with a Prostate-Specific Antigen Level < 4.0 ng per Milliliter." *New England Journal of Medicine* 24 (2004): 2239–46.

Warlick, Christopher, Bruce J. Trock, and others. "Delayed Versus Immediate Surgical Intervention and Prostate Cancer Outcome." *Journal of the National Cancer Institute* 98 (2006): 355–57.

CHAPTER FIVE

Brokaw, Tom. *The Greatest Generation Speaks: Letters and Reflections.* New York: Random House, 2005.

Hallerman, Victoria. *How We Survived Prostate Cancer: What We Did and What We Should Have Done.* New York: Newmarket Press, 2009.

King, Larry. Interview with Tom Brokaw. Aired March 6, 2000.

Living With Prostate Cancer: A Wife's Passion website, 2011. Available at http://prostatecancerblog.net/. Accessed October 2011.

The Memorial Sloan-Kettering Cancer Center website, 2011. Available at http://www.mskcc.org/mskcc/html/44.cfm. Accessed October 2011.

CHAPTER SIX

Medical News Today website, 2011. Available at www.medicalnewstoday.com. Accessed October 2011.

National Cancer Institute website, 2011. Available at www.cancer.gov. Accessed October 2011.

US National Library of Medicine website, 2011. Available at http://www.ncbi.nlm.nih.gov/pubmed. Accessed October 2011.

CHAPTER SEVEN

New York Times (New York) 8 July 2009.

"Prostate Cancer Drug Discoveries: What the Future Holds." Market Report: Espicom Business Intelligence, May 31, 2007.

"Prostate Cancer Therapeutics: A Global Strategic Business Report." Press Release: Global Industry Analysts, April 6, 2009.

Smith, Benjamin, Grace L. Smith, and others. "Future of Cancer Incidence in the United States: Burdens Upon an Aging, Changing Nation." *Journal of Clinical Oncology* 27 (September 2009): 2758–765.

Snyder, C.F., K.D. Frick, and others. "Costs of Treatments for Local/Regional Prostate Cancer." *Journal of Clinical Oncology* 27 (2009): suppl, abstr 6527.

The Surveillance Epidemiology and End Results (SEER) Database, National Cancer Institute, National Institutes of Health website, 2009. Available at www.seer.cancer.gov. Accessed July 2009.

Thompson, Mary, and Robert Neil. "Prostate Cancer Market: $2 Billion and Growing." Medtech Insight: FDC-Windhover Information, February 2008.

Wilson, L.S., R. Tesoro, and others. "Cumulative Cost Pattern Comparison of Prostate Cancer Treatment." *Cancer* 109 (2007): 518–27.

CHAPTER EIGHT

Blute, Michael L. "No Proof of Inferiority: Open Radical Retropubic Prostatectomy Remains State-of-the-Art Surgical Technique for Localized Prostate Cancer." *The Journal of Urology* 181 (June 2009): 2421–423.

Efstathiou, Jason A., Alexei V. Trofimov, and Anthony L. Zeitman. "Life, Liberty, and the Pursuit of Protons: An Evidence-Based Review of the Role of Particle Therapy in the Treatment of Prostate Cancer." *The Cancer Journal* 15 (July/August 2009): 312–18.

Friedlander, Terence W., and Charles J. Ryan. "Novel Hormonal Approaches in Prostate Cancer." *Current Oncology Reports* 11 (2009): 227–34.

Global Information, Inc. website, 2011. Available at http://www. giiresearch.com. Accessed November 2011.

Isbarn, H., L. Boccon-Gibod, and others. "Androgen Deprivation Therapy for the Treatment of Prostate Cancer: Consider both Benefits and Risks." *European Urology* 55 (2009): 62–75.

Konski, A. A. "Intensity-Modulated Radiation Therapy is a Cost-Effective Treatment for Intermediate-Risk Prostate Cancer." ASTRO Presentation, 2004. Abstract 26.

Konski, A.A., W. Speier, and others. "Is Proton Beam Therapy Cost Effective in the Treatment of Adenocarcinoma of the Prostate?" *Journal of Clinical Oncology* 25 (2007): 3603–308.

Kuban, Deborah A. "Localized Prostate Cancer: The Battle of Treatment Options Enters the Larger Arena." *Oncology* 23 (14 September 2009): 867, 873.

Pruthi, Raj S., and Eric M. Wallen. "Current Status of Robotic Prostatectomy: Promises Fulfilled." *The Journal of Urology* 181 (June 2009); 2420–421.

Rayala, Heidi J., and Jerome P. Richie. "Radical Prostatectomy Reigns Supreme." *Oncology* 23 (14 September 2009): Available at http://www.cancernetwork.com/display/article/10165/1453623 Accessed December 2011.

Saylor, Philip J., and Matthew R. Smith. "Metabolic Complications of Androgen Deprivation Therapy for Prostate Cancer." *The Journal of Urology* 181 (2009): 1998–2008.

Senior Journal website, 2011. Available at www.seniorjournal.com. Accessed November 2011.

The New York Times (New York) 1 December 2006.

Whelan, David, and Robert Langreth. "The $150 Million Zapper." *Forbes* (16 March 2009): 62–3.

Zeitman, Anthony L. "The Titantic and the Iceberg: Prostate Proton Therapy and Health Care Economics." *Journal of Clinical Oncology* 25 (2007): 3565–566.

CHAPTER NINE

American Prostate Society website http://www.american prostatesociety.com/ Accessed December 2011.

Barbara Ehrenreich, "Cancerland," *Harper's Magazine*, November 2001

Congressionally Directed Medical Research programs (CDMRP) website http://cdmrp.army.mil/default.shtml Accessed December 2011.

Haran C. Vince DeVita: "The view from the top." *Cancer World* June–July 2005; 38–43.

Karen M. Kedrowski and Marilyn Stine Sarow, *Cancer Activism: Gender, Media, and Public Policy* Urbana: University of Illinois Press, 2007

National Breast Cancer Coalition website. http://www.breast cancerdeadline2020.org/about/history/ Accessed December 2011.

National Cancer Institute website (cancer.gov) http://www.cancer. gov/cancertopics/types/prostate Accessed November 2011 ; http://www.cancer.gov/cancertopics/types/breast Accessed November 2011.

New York Times (New York) "The Year of the Ribbon." May 5, 1992.

Patient Advocates for Advanced Cancer Treatment website http:// www.paactusa.org/ Accessed December 2011.

Prostate Cancer Conditions Education Council website http:// www.prostateconditions.org/ Accessed December 2011.

Susan G. Komen Foundation website http://ww5.komen.org/mil-liondollarcouncil.aspx Accessed December 2011. http://ww5. komen.org/AboutUs/AboutUs.html Accessed December 2011.

Suzanne Fletcher, 1997. "Whither Scientific Deliberation in Health Policy Recommendations? Alice in the Wonderland of Breast Cancer Screening." *New England Journal of Medicine* 336(16): 1180–83

Tara Parker-Hope, "Cancer Funding: Does It Add Up?" New York: *New York Times*, March 6, 2008.

The Breast Cancer Research Foundation http://www.bcrfcure.org/ about_history.html Accessed December 2011.

The Surveillance Epidemiology and End Results (SEER) Database, National Cancer Institute, National Institutes of Health website, http://seer.cancer.gov/csr/1975_2005/results_sin-gle/sect_01_table.01.pdf Accessed March 2010.

CHAPTER TEN

Ben Witherington's website, 2011. Available at www.benwith erington.blogspot.com. Accessed March 2009.

Chambers, Oswald. *My Utmost for His Highest*. Grand Rapids, Mich: Discovery House Publishers, 2008.

Nepo, Mark. "God, Self, and Medicine." *The Patient's Voice: Experiences of Illness*, ed. Jeaninne Young-Mason. Philidelphia: F. A. Davis, 1997.

Stuntz, William. "Three Gifts for Hard Times." *Christianity Today* (August 2009): Available at http://www.christianity today. com/ct/2009/august/34.44.html Accessed December 2011.

Wohlbrecht, Sara. "The Triangle: In." Sermon delivered at Saint Matthew Lutheran Church. Walnut Creek, California (March 15, 2009).

Wright, N. T. "Kingdom Come: The Public Meaning of the Gospels." *Christian Century* (June 17, 2008): Available at http://cruciality. wordpress.com/2008/06/17/nt-wright-kingdom-come-the-public-meaning-of-the-gospels/ Accessed December 2011.

Wright, N. T. *Surprised by Hope*. New York: Harper One, 2008.

CHAPTER ELEVEN

Antonelli, J., S. J. Freedland, and L. W. Jones. "Exercise Therapy Across the Prostate Cancer Continuum." *Prostate Cancer and Prostatic Diseases* 12 (2009): 110–15.

Chan, June M., Crystal N. Holick, and others. "Diet after Diagnosis and the Risk of Prostate Cancer Progression, Recurrence, and Death (United States)." *Cancer Causes and Control* 17 (2006): 199–208.

Chan, June M., Peter H. Gann, and Edward L. Giovannucci. "Role of Diet in Prostate Cancer Development and Progression." *Journal of Clinical Oncology* 23 (November 10, 2005): 8152–160.

Couper, Jeremy W. "The Effects of Prostate Cancer on Intimate Relationships." *Journal of Men's Health and Gender* 4 (September 2007): 226–32.

Cushman, Mitchell A., JoAnne L. Phillips, and Richard J. Wassersug. "The Language of Emasculation: Implications for Cancer Patients." *International Journal of Men's Health* 9 (Spring 2010): 3–25.

Efstathiou, J. A., B. Kyounghwa, and others. "Obesity and Mortality in Men with Locally Advanced Prostate Cancer." *Cancer* 110 (December 15 2007): 2691–699.

Herr, Harry W., and Maryellen O'Sullivan. "Quality of Life of Asymptomatic Men with Nonmetastatic Prostate Cancer on Androgen Deprivation Therapy." *The Journal of Urology* 163 (June 2000): 1743–746.

Navon, Liora, and Amira Morag. "Advanced Prostate Cancer Patients' Ways of Coping with the Hormonal Therapy's Effect on Body, Sexuality, and Spousal Ties." *Qualitative Health Research* 13 (2003): 1378–392.

Segal, Roanne J., Robert D. Reid, and others. "Resistance Exercise in Men Receiving Androgen Deprivation Therapy for Prostate Cancer." *Journal of Clinical Oncology* 21 (May 1, 2003): 1653–659.

Wassersug, Richard J. "Mastering Emasculation." *Journal of Clinical Oncology* 27 (February 1, 2009): 634–36.

EPILOGUE

Andriole, Gerald L., E. David Crawford, and others. "Mortality Results from a Randomized Prostate-Cancer Screening Trial." *New England Journal of Medicine* 360 (March 26, 2009): 1320–328.

Daniels, Kaer, Graves Kim, and others. "Implantable Device for Cancer Monitoring." *Biosensors and Bioelectronics* 24 (July 15, 2009): 3252–257.

Laxman, Bharathi, David S. Morris, and others. "A First-Generation Multiplex Biomarker Analysis of Urine for the Early Detection of Prostate Cancer." *Cancer Research* 68 (February 1, 2008): 645.

"The Man Who Changed Medicine." *Fortune Magazine* (November 29, 2004): Available at http://money.cnn.com/magazines/fortune/fortune_archive/2004/11/29/8192713/index.htm Accessed December 2011.

Scales, Charles D., Jr., Judd W. Moul, and others. "Prostate Cancer in the Baby Boomer Generation: Results from CaPSURE." *Urology* 70 (2007): 1162–167.

Schroder, Fritz H., Jonas Hugosson, and others. "Screening and Prostate-Cancer Mortality in a Randomized European Study." *New England Journal of Medicine* 360 (March 26, 2009): 1320–328.

Smith, Benjamin D., Grace L. Smith, and others. "Future of Cancer Incidence in the United States: Burdens Upon an Aging, Changing Nation." *Journal of Clinical Oncology* 27 (June 2009): 2758–765.

Sullivan, Andrew. "Goodbye to All That: Why Obama Matters." *The Atlantic* (December 2007): Available at http://www.theatlantic.com/magazine/archive/2007/12/goodbye-to-all-that-why-obama-matters/6445/ Accessed December 2011.

U.S. Mintel International Group, Ltd. *Baby Boomers and Health.* May 1, 2004.

Index

AAM, *See* Anti-androgen
  monotherapy
ACS, *See* American Cancer
  Society
Active surveillance, *See* Expectant
  management
Adenocarcinoma, 18, 19
ADT, *See* Androgen deprivation
  therapy
AIDS, 174
  advocacy groups, 152, 153
American Cancer Society (ACS),
  47, 66, 95
American medical system, 72
Androgen deprivation therapy
  (ADT), 30, 36, 37, 43, 120,
  122, 132, 133, 188, 190,
  202, 203
  bone-weakening effects of, 197
  clinical goal of, 187
  complications of, 193
  effects, 201
  side effects, 91–93
  treatments, 92

Androgen receptors, 30, 37
Androgen suppression, 95
  drugs, side effects of, 193
Annealing treatment process,
  204–205
Anti-androgen, 30
  drugs, 94, 96
    ADT, 93
    radiotherapy, 92, 95
  medication, 52, 53, 54, 61
Anti-androgen monotherapy
  (AAM), 132
Autologous cellular immunother-
  apy, 134
Awareness ribbons, 152

Benign prostatic hyperplasia
  (BPH), 22
Bicalutamide, *See* Casodex®
Biopsy
  needle, 9, 63
  prostate, 9
  reflections on, 17–20
  urethral, 51, 53, 55, 60

Body Mass Index (BMI), 192
Bone scan, 52, 54, 61
Bone-weakening effects
    of ADT, 197
Bowel irregularity, 119
BPH, *See* Benign prostatic
    hyperplasia
BrainLab, 143, 145
Breast cancer, 200, 203
    advocacy
        biopsy for, 154, 155
        pink ribbons, 153–158

Cancer
    cells, 36, 186
    staging, 62
    type of, 12
Cancer Activism, 156, 160
Carcinogen, 13
Casodex®, 37
Castrate-resistant prostate cancer
    (CRPC), 133, 189
CCC, *See* Cumulative Cost
    Comparison of Prostate
    Cancer Treatments
CDMRP, *See* Congressionally
    Directed Medical Research
    Program
Cells, cancer, 36, 186
Cellular immunotherapy, autolo-
    gous, 134
Chemical castration, 71
Chemotherapy, 59, 65, 66, 73, 85,
    133, 134
Chronic pain, 173
Chronic prostatitis, 24
Colon cancer, 173
Combat ribbons, 152–153
Combined androgen blockade
    (CAB), 188, 200
Communication, 69–70
    about cancer, 74
    social networking, 81
    target audiences, 82
    writing, 83

Community support to patient,
    167–170
Congressionally Directed Medical
    Research Program
    (CDMRP), 157, 160, 163
CRPC, *See* Castrate-resistant
    prostate cancer
CT scan, 6, 7, 77, 101, 102
Cultural silence, 70–71
Cumulative Cost Comparison
    of Prostate Cancer
    Treatments, 123, 125, 126
Cystoscopy, 10

Death rate in prostate cancer, 114
Diagnostic code 185, 35–39
Diet, 192–198
Digital rectal exam (DRE), 8, 30,
    41–42, 173

EBRT, *See* Electron beam
    radiotherapy
ED, *See* Erectile dysfunction
Electron beam radiotherapy
    (EBRT), 74, 136, 138
Emergency room (ER), 5–7, 150
Erectile dysfunction (ED), 72
Ethnicity, prostate cancer
    mortality rates by, 114
Exercise and diet, 192–198
Expectant management, 32,
    64, 120
External beam radiation therapy
    (EBRT), 28

Fatigue, 79

Genitourinary history, 20–22
Genotypes, 189
Gleason scoring system, 36, 45, 46,
    53, 64, 65
Gonadotropin releasing hormone
    (GnRH), 29
Grassroots survivor organizations
    (GSOs), 156, 160

Halstead mastectomy, 154
HDR, *See* High dose rate
    brachytherapy
Healing, problem of prayers for,
    181–183
Hematuria, 172
High dose rate (HDR)
    brachytherapy, 127
Hitchhiker's Guide to the Galaxy
    (Adams), 173
Hormone ablation, 28
Hormone treatment (HT), 30, 33,
    59, 61, 67, 71, 75, 97–98,
    187, 194, 197
Hydrocortisone, 189

Image-guided radiotherapy (IGRT),
    33, 75, 136, 137, 138
Immunotherapy, 59
    autologous cellular, 134
IMRT, *See* Intensity-modulated
    radiotherapy
Indolent cancers, 126
Intensity-modulated radiotherapy
    (IMRT), 33, 75, 76, 136, 137,
    138, 142
International Classification of
    Diseases (ICD9), 40
Internet, cancer research tool, 94–97

Journal of Urology, 72

Ketoconazole, 133, 189

LHRH, *See* Luteinizing hormone-
    releasing hormone
Lidocaine, 98
Light blue ribbons for prostate
    cancer advocacy, 158–162
Localized prostate cancer, 115, 116,
    122, 129, 131
Lung cancer, 163
Lupron®, 102
Luteinizing hormone-releasing
    hormone (LHRH), 29

Medicare reimbursement, 141
Member Organizations of
    the Prostate Cancer
    Roundtable, 161
Metamorphosis, 38
Metaphor, apt, 35
Microsurgery, 67
Morphine-based painkiller, 56
MRI scan, 99
Multiple sclerosis (MS), 79–80

National Breast Cancer Awareness
    Month (NBCAM), 155
National Breast Cancer Coalition
    (NBCC), 157
National Cancer Institute
    (NCI), 93, 95, 162, 163
    website, 55
National Defense Service
    Medal, 152
National Prostate Cancer Coalition
    (NPCC), 159
Navy Achievement Medal, 152
NBCAM, *See* National Breast
    Cancer Awareness Month
NBCC, *See* National Breast Cancer
    Coalition
NCI, *See* National Cancer
    Institute
Needle biopsy, 9, 63
Nerve-sparing surgery, 59
Nerve-sparing technique, 129
Nomograms, 75, 99
Novalis treatment, 142–146, 151
NPCC, *See* National Prostate
    Cancer Coalition

Oncologists, 14
Oncology Adventure Ride, 93, 113,
    119, 120, 151
Open RP, *See* Radical retropubic
    prostatectomy
Osteopenia, bone, 54
Osteoporosis, 193
    bone, 54

Patient couch, 111
PBRT, *See* Proton beam
    radiotherapy
PCEC, *See* Prostate Cancer
    Education Council
PCF, *See* Prostate Cancer
    Foundation
Pharmaceuticals, 132–136
PIN, *See* Prostatic interepithelial
    neoplasia; Prostatic
    intraepithelial neoplasia
Pink ribbons for breast cancer
    advocacy, 153–158
PRBT, *See* Proton beam
    radiotherapy
Primus, 110, 112, 113, 118–120, 142,
    144
Prostate biopsy, 9
Prostate cancer
    advocacy, 156, 160, 164
        light blue ribbons, 158–162
    causes of, 23–25, 117
    curative trail, 185–192
    diagnosis of, 52
    history of, 25–34
    side effects of, 15
    survey of, 14
    treatment community, 188
Prostate Cancer Education Council
    (PCEC), 159
Prostate Cancer Foundation (PCF),
    154, 159, 162
Prostate cancer treatment market
    death rate in, 114
    dimensions of, 113–116
    stage distribution, 115
    survival rate, 116
Prostate cells, 9
Prostate-specific antigen (PSA), 8,
    21, 30–33, 42, 46, 187
    screening, 115, 124
    test, 158, 173
Prostate tumors, 115
Prostatic interepithelial neoplasia
    (PIN), 22, 38

Prostatitis, 22
Proton beam radiotherapy (PBRT),
    33, 76–77, 122, 136,
    138–139
Provenge ®, 189
PSA, *See* Prostate-specific antigen

Radiation, 147–152, 185, 186, 188
Radiation oncology, 74–78
Radiation Oncology Center, 63, 109,
    142, 150, 151
    treatment table in, 113
Radical prostatectomy (RP), 129
Radical retropubic prostatectomy
    (RRP), 130
Radioactive needles, 67
Radiotherapy, 59, 68, 75, 76, 97, 101,
    104, 127, 129, 143, 148, 152,
    168, 186
    ADT, 95
    preparation for, 102
    side effects of, 120
    x-rays, 97
RALP, *See* Robot assisted laparo-
    scopic prostatectomy
Reclast®, 192
Relationship with cancer, 57–60,
    67, 69
Responses of family, 86–90
Robot assisted laparoscopic
    prostatectomy (RALP), 130
Robotic approach, 130, 131
Robotic prostatectomy, 109
RP, *See* Radical prostatectomy
RRP, *See* Radical retropubic
    prostatectomy

SEER, *See* Surveillance
    Epidemiology and End
    Results database
Sexist claims, 190
Siemens Primus linear accelerator,
    See Primus
Surgery, 59–60, 129–132
Surprised by Hope (Wright), 178